LAW EVERY NURSE SHOULD KNOW

Second Edition

HELEN CREIGHTON, R.N., B.S.N., A.B., A.M., M.S.N., J.D.

Professor of Nursing, University of Wisconsin-Milwaukee,
Milwaukee, Wisconsin

W. B. SAUNDERS COMPANY • PHILADELPHIA • LONDON • TORONTO

W. B. Saunders Company: West Washington Square
                         Philadelphia, Pa. 19105

                         12 Dyott Street
                         London, WC1A 1DB

                         1835 Yonge Street
                         Toronto 7, Ontario

Law Every Nurse Should Know   SBN 0-7216-2751-X

Print No.:   9   8   7   6   5   4

Preface

In an age which gives great emphasis to the legal rights of people, the revised edition of this handbook is designed to present nurses with the basic facts of law in a concise, nontechnical manner. It is intended so to acquaint the nurse with her rights and duties at law that in her work she will conduct herself as an ordinary, reasonable nurse, and will do so with greater ease and comfort. The nurse's license to practice as a registered professional nurse with or without specialization or as a practical nurse means more to the nurse who understands the purpose and problems of licensure. The nurse who knows her contractual rights, duties and remedies is likely to make better and breach fewer contracts. Recent cases as well as older cases involving nurses in negligence and malpractice suits show how such problems can and do arise. The legal status of a nurse in today's changed and changing world and her liabilities and rights in relation to various paying positions are discussed. How and why suits for such wrongs as assault and battery, false imprisonment, invasion of the right of privacy, and defamation of character originate are illustrated. Such of the crimes, great and small, as a nurse seems most likely to encounter are presented. The impact of newer legislation, such as good samaritan laws and child abuse laws, is discussed. Many new topics are presented; among them are telephone orders; paramedical personnel: aides, orderlies and attendants; closed chest cardio-pulmonary resuscitation; the role of the nurse in acute cardiac care; sterilization; and transplantation of organs. Some pertinent information on the topics of witnesses and wills increase the nurse's general knowledge and help her to meet emergency situations.

At the end of Chapters 2 through 11, the reader will find a number of references which will enable her to pursue points of interest in greater depth. These references will be particularly useful and time-saving for students and others who need additional material and who have limited time to review available literature.

Any person who writes a book is indebted to others for a great deal of useful assistance and encouragement. In particular, I wish to express my appreciation to the following: my mother, Mrs. Helen Miller Creighton Reitz; Sister Catherine Armington, D.C., Health Coordinator, Marillac College, St. Louis; Sister Angela Marie Carrico, S.C.N., former Dean of Georgetown University School of Nursing and now Associate Director of Nursing Services and Director of In-Service Education, Methodist Hospital, Henderson, Kentucky; Mrs. Ruby Tillery, Dean, University of Southwestern Louisiana; Mrs. Carrie Sutherlin Montz, retired junior college president, and her husband, John Montz, now at Wesley Woods Towers, Atlanta, Georgia; Ann B. Vose, Director of Nursing, the Nursing Service Advisory Council, the Nursing Care Advisors and the Library Staff of 1968–1969 at Barnes Hospital in St. Louis; Constance V. S. Wilson, R.N., retired, Washington, D.C.; Sister Gabriella Richard, D.C., Nurse-Supervisor, United States Public Health Hospital, Carville, Louisiana; Dr. William P. Argy, Fellow in Internal Medicine, and Dr. Gerald McAteer, Surgeon, both of Washington, D.C.; and the many unnamed Daughters of Charity throughout the central and southern United States and the Carmelites of Lafayette for many acts of kindness and support. I thank all those who have attended my lectures, workshops and classes for their questions and encouragement.

Finally, I am grateful to Dr. Inez G. Hinsvark, Dean of the School of Nursing at the University of Wisconsin–Milwaukee, for the freedom she gives coworkers in daily operations, her generous support, her recognition of their efforts and her unfailing habit of extending to each person a feeling that he or she has much worth.

HELEN CREIGHTON

Contents

Chapter Six

The Relation of a Nurse's Rights and Liabilities to Her
Position and Status 73

Chapter Seven

Chapter Eight

Chapter Nine

CRIMES: MISDEMEANORS AND FELONIES 169

Chapter One

Law and Society

ORIGIN OF COMMON LAW AND CIVIL LAW

The earliest notion of law was not a declaration or decree of a legislative or executive agency. In the early ages, law was the pronouncement of the king, or some other ruler, acting according to what was thought to be his "divine right." A body of law developed from an accumulation of judgments arising from particular cases. This practice of building a system of rules and sanctions by the accumulation of case-to-case decisions has remained to this day the unique characteristic of Anglo-American jurisprudence. The body of case law which developed from the adjudications of kings, and later of judges, is known as "the common law." The common law, or judge-made law, is to be contrasted with the law emanating from legislative bodies such as Parliament, Congress or city councils; the law coming from such bodies is civil law, also known as positive law. The law in force today in the United States is a combination of both the common law and legislation, the latter increasing in importance and quantity each year.

The fundamental principles which have guided the growth of American law had their origin in England. As already noted, the king asserted absolute power to dictate the standards of social conduct among his subjects. This power was steadily diminished by demands

1

of influential nobles that the judgment of the monarch be guided by the customs and traditions of his people. Indeed, certain areas of life were placed beyond the reach of the Crown. In 1215, the famous *Magna Charta* was granted by King John of England, and came to be known as the foundation of English constitutional liberty. This landmark in the struggle of human freedom is significant in that it placed effective restraints upon the exercise of governmental power and at the same time secured the personal liberty of the subject and his rights to property. Thus, law has a dual function: to confirm certain rights and privileges in the person with means for their enforcement, and to provide a framework of government, together with its powers and restrictions upon the exercise of those powers.

DEFINITION OF LAW

At this point, it is instructive to look more closely at the terms "law" and "law of the land." The terms are generalizations and, as may be readily understood, do not lend themselves to precise definition. A workable definition of the term "law" would be: those standards of human conduct established and enforced by the authority of an organized society through its government. Law is not synonymous with custom, although custom plays an important role in creating and enforcing law. Indeed, there are areas of life wherein custom is a much more powerful dictate of human conduct than the law enforced by the state. But the point to be emphasized is that there is no law, in the sense that the term is used here, apart from a government which ordains and enforces the command.

FORM OF GOVERNMENT IN THE UNITED STATES

The three levels of government in the United States, federal, state and local, are created by law and in turn exercise powers derived from law. Thus it is said that Americans live under a "government of law, not of men." This means that before the government may act, it must find some authority for that act in law. The law may take the form of a constitution, a statute, an administrative regulation or a court decision interpreting these forms of law. Hence, the expression "law of the land" means that every citizen shall hold his life, liberty, property and immunities under the protection of general rules which govern society. Furthermore, these rights may not be properly infringed upon unless there has been a proceeding conforming to the law, that is to say, a hearing and inquiry before judgment is rendered at trial.

Federal Constitution and Federal Government

The highest form of law in the United States is the Constitution. The Federal Constitution is known as the "organic law"; that is to say, it is law which defines or establishes the very organization of the government. The Constitution provides for the framework of the Federal Government in establishing the three branches, Legislative, Executive and Judicial. The instrument also clothes these branches of government with powers to act and at the same time places restraints upon the exercise of those powers.

State Constitutions and State Government

In addition to the Federal Government, every state has a constitution. A significant difference in function should be noted: namely, the only powers which the Federal Government enjoys are derived from the positive grants of power of the Federal Constitution, while the state governments enjoy plenary powers subject only to the limitations of the state constitutions, the limitations upon states found in the Federal Constitution, and those limitations necessary for the operation of the federal system.

Local and City Governments

Lastly, local governments are creatures of the states which created them and may exercise only those powers conferred upon them.

STATUTORY LAW

When Congress exercises the legislative powers conferred by the Federal Constitution, its enactments are known as statutory law. When a state legislature enacts a law, it is similarly described. Publications containing statutes are referred to as codes. Thus, the Federal statutes are contained in the United States Code, and those of the various states are contained in similar compilations. The product of law-making power by a city council is known as a city ordinance.

Administrative Law

Since the turn of the century, another branch of public law has become of great importance, that is, administrative law. One may readily understand that when Congress or a state legislature desires to enact a program of regulation of business, or a program to confer benefits upon its citizens, it is difficult for the legislature to foresee the variations necessary for the proper execution of the law. The legislature lacks the time and energy to include all the many details likely to arise when the law is put into operation. The legislature, by way of providing for these eventualities, establishes an administrative agency clothed with power to make rules and regulations which have the force of law. The administrative agencies may also issue orders which have the effect of a court order to take care of violations of its rules and regulations. Actions of the agencies are appealable to the courts. The Interstate Commerce Commission on the Federal level and a bureau of conservation on a state level are examples of administrative agencies.

Public law.   In the preceding paragraph, the term "public law" was used. *Public law* is that branch of law concerned with the state in its political capacity and includes, as noted, constitutional and administrative law. The relationship of the individual or individuals to the state is included in public law, the most striking example of which occurs in enforcement of criminal law.

Criminal Law.   More particularly, *criminal law* deals with acts or offenses against the welfare or safety of the public.

Private law.   By contrast, *private law* refers to that part of the law which is administered between citizen and citizen, or is concerned with the enforcement of rights, duties and other legal relations involving private individuals. The law of contract, of negligence and of agent-principal dealings are areas of private law.

Equity.   While the common law system of justice was developing in England, another field of jurisdiction, known as *equity*, was growing up beside it. When the application of the civil law became too harsh or when there was no adequate remedy in the common law to satisfy the needs of a petitioner, an appeal was taken to the king. The appeal was made to "conscience," that is to say, to the king's innate sense of justice and right. If the king were convinced that an exception to the common law should be made in the case before him, he would so order. Gradually, separate tribunals were set up, known as courts of chancery (because the king appointed a substitute, known as a chancellor, to hear such matters) or courts of equity. Equity developed its own set of principles, rules and precedents, and when these clashed with their counterparts in the common law courts, equity was held to prevail. Equity, it was said, acted in accordance with the spirit, not the letter, of the law. It played and continues to play an important role in the operation of the American judicial system.

STRUCTURE OF AMERICAN GOVERNMENT

The functioning of any system of law is affected by the form of government. The countries of the world today are organized according to either a unitary (also known as centralized) or a federal form of government. In a unitary state, all governmental powers are vested in the central government, as provided in its constitution, and no subdivisions exist as independent political units. The central government may allocate certain functions to subsidiary units, but such functions are exercised solely by the grace and sufferance of the central power. The United Kingdom, France, Belgium and many other European countries are unitary states. In a federal system, the people are not placed under a single government endowed with full powers exercised from one center. There is a spatial or territorial division of governmental power between the central, or national, government and the constituent units. In the United States, the constituent units are known as states, in Canada as provinces, and in Switzerland as cantons. All these countries and many more are federal in form. The powers of government are divided, some exclusively exercised by the federal or national government, and others exclusively exercised by the state governments.

Powers of Federal and State Governments

The significant fact to note in a federal form of government is that the constituent units are separate and, to a considerable extent, independent political powers. Under the Federal Constitution, the states retain for themselves all powers not specifically conferred upon the Federal Government. Because of the division of governmental power among various jurisdictions within a federal system, laws differ from state to state. Moreover, since there are two sovereigns in a federal system, a conviction under the laws of one (say, the Federal Government) does not preclude a conviction under the laws of the other (state laws) for the same offense. Finally, some powers may be exercised by both the federal and the state governments. These powers are called "concurrent powers."

Doctrine of Separation of Powers

The sovereign powers in the United States are not only divided according to territory, that is, federalized, but they are also divided internally. This internal division of power is referred to as the doctrine of separation of powers. Recalling the evils of absolutism in the English experience, the founders of the American government were guided by the truism that "power corrupts and absolute power corrupts absolutely." They believed that one person or one branch of the government should not enjoy all the power, but that it should be divided so that one branch could serve as a check upon another.

Legislative, administrative, judiciary. Consequently, the law-making power is conferred upon the Congress, but the Executive can veto legislation, and the Judiciary is empowered to review legislation. Likewise, Congress could withhold funds from, and investigate, the Executive and control the appellate jurisdiction of the federal courts.

Subdivisions of States

As was noted in a preceding paragraph, the third level of government in the United States, municipalities, arises from the power of states to create political subdivisions. These units of local government include counties, cities, towns, townships, boroughs and villages. The designation of a local community may not be indicative of its size. That is to say, there are townships with populations larger than some cities, but since the township has not been chartered by the state as a city it may not use the latter designation. States confer powers upon their subdivisions to make local laws or ordinances, which are operative only within the geographical boundaries of the local communities. Though the Federal Government is powerless to abolish a state by its own act, a state may rescind a charter it had granted to a city and govern the city directly from the state capital. There is no provision in the Federal Constitution about the relationship of the states and their subdivisions.

SOURCES OF LAW

In the foregoing pages of this chapter, the general nature of law and the structure of American government have been described. It is now desirable to review some of the sources of law and the principles which guide courts in their output of decisional law.

Statutory Law

Statutory law, as has been noted, is that law enacted by a legislative body, such as Congress. After enactment, Federal laws are published in the *United States Statutes at Large.* The original copy of the act, with the President's signature, is filed or deposited with the government agency responsible for its administration or enforcement. For example, a pure food law is administered by the Department of Agriculture; a law relating to the national parks is sent to the

Department of the Interior. As for acts of state legislatures, copies are deposited with the secretary of state of the state. Municipal ordinances are deposited with local authorities. The public generally receives notice of legislation from the daily press and other communication media.

Decisional Law

In addition to statute law, another important source of law is decisional law, or the law announced when courts rule on cases brought before them.

COURTS

Courts are agencies established by the government to decide disputes arising in litigation. The term "court" may be used in another sense as referring to the person or persons hearing the case. More particularly, the court may consist of the judge, the magistrate or the justice. At trials, usually only one judge sits; when cases are taken to courts of appeal, more than one judge hears the appeal.

Criminal Court, Civil Court, Probate Court

The kind of court in which a case is brought depends upon the offense or complaint involved. For example, the proceeding is handled in a criminal court if it involves a traffic violation or the unlawful killing of a person. A claim for damages, by contrast, is a dispute as to the legal rights and duties of individuals in relation to each other, and is known as a civil action. Actions concerning wills or the estates of decedents are known as probate proceedings and, as civil cases, may be heard in courts of general jurisdiction or, in some states, in courts known as surrogate or orphans courts.

Jurisdiction of Courts

There are certain legal principles which guide courts in deciding disputes. First, the court must have jurisdiction over the person or the thing involved. This means that the proceeding is commenced in a court in the locality in which the defendant resides or may be served with a summons, or in which the property is situated.

The United States District Courts have original jurisdiction over admiralty cases, bankruptcy cases, postal and banking law cases and crimes involving Federal laws or those committed on the high seas. In addition, they have jurisdiction over cases involving a question of the

Constitution, a treaty, a Federal law or a lawsuit between citizens of different states or between the United States and a state if the amount involved is not in excess of $3000.

The Supreme Court of the United States has original jurisdiction over cases involving ambassadors, public ministers and consuls and in lawsuits in which the state is a party and the amount involved is over $3000. However, the bulk of its work consists of hearing appeals from the decisions of the circuit court of appeals. A case which involves a constitutional question may be heard directly from the United States District Courts. Cases from state courts which involve the United States Constitution or the constitutionality of any state or Federal law may be brought to the Supreme Court either directly or on appeal.

Since our social and economic systems have become increasingly complex, and with the explosion of knowledge in all fields, it is not possible to include within the statutes sufficient detail to cover adequately all situations that may arise in the practical application of the intent of the law. Hence, the Government has established on a statutory basis a large and ever-increasing number of Federal administrative agencies for the purpose of implementing the intent of legislation. The administrative agency has the power and responsibility to make whatever rules, regulations and standards are necessary to carry out the purpose of the law. However, such powers and responsibilities must be in conformity with existing laws. Several examples of Federal administrative agencies are the Federal Trade Commission, the Social Security Board, the Federal Communications Commission, the National Labor Relations Board and the Interstate Commerce Commission.

The United States is immune from suit unless Congress gives authority otherwise, such as by a private bill device in an individual case or by an act such as The Federal Tort Claims Act. Moreover, the state, which is also a sovereign body, may not be sued without its own consent.

In most states, there are county courts which try both civil and criminal cases arising within the county. Usually, there is a limit on the amount of money damages which can be sought in this court.

In villages, towns and rural areas, there are Justice of the Peace Courts. They are a part of the state judicial system and may hear civil cases involving small sums of money, try those charged with misdemeanors and conduct a preliminary examination of those accused of felonies.

Generally, state superior courts have only appellate jurisdiction. They are variously called, in different states, circuit courts, supreme courts, district courts or courts of common pleas.

Every state has a final court of appeals. Again, its name varies from state to state. While it is often called the Supreme Court, it may also be known as the Supreme Court of Errors, the Court of Appeals or the Supreme Judicial Court.

State legislatures, following the pattern of the Federal Government, have created a variety of boards, commissions and administrative agencies to deal with much of the work. Their proceedings are informal and they are not bound by the rules of evidence. Two examples of such agencies are the Public Service Commission and the Workmen's Compensation Board.

Stare Decisis

The second principle by which courts are guided is known as *stare decisis,* which is to say, "the previous decision stands." When a previous case involving similar facts has been decided in the jurisdiction, the court will be strongly inclined to follow the principle of law laid down in that prior adjudication. Unless precedents are carefully regarded and adhered to, uncertainty would be both perplexing and prejudicial to the public. However, when the precedent is out of date, or inapplicable to the case before the court, the principle of *stare decisis* will not be followed and the court will announce a new rule.

HOW LAWS ARE RECORDED

Judicial opinions of federal and state appellate courts are published, but those of trial courts are generally unavailable in this form. By an elaborate system of references and indexes, the many thousands of decisions are kept up-to-date for research and current use.

Chapter Two

The Practice of Nursing

HISTORY OF THE PROFESSION OF NURSING

The profession of nursing has progressed a long way since the time that Florence Nightingale was able to have it recognized as a secular occupation which requires skill and training by which a person may gain a livelihood.

Although there are still problems to be worked out to improve the legal position of the profession, much beneficial legislation has been enacted as a result of the efforts of a group of unusually sincere, energetic, public-spirited members of the nursing profession. The existing law leaves certain things to be desired, including changes in the following areas: a clear definition of nursing practice, more adequate control by the state board of nurses' examiners, the qualifications of members of the state nursing board commensurate with the profession's ability to give its best service to the public, flexibility in interstate licensing, and mandatory licensing in all jurisdictions. As might be expected in our system of states' rights, there is a lack of uniformity from jurisdiction to jurisdiction, but hope for further improvement lies in the continued efforts of the zealous group of nurses ever at work in the interest of the profession. A considerable amount of progress has been already accomplished through the concerted action of various associations, notably the American Nurses' Association, the National League for Nursing, and other national associations. Schools of nursing and the efforts of individuals have added to the ever-continuing march of progress.

DEFINITION OF LICENSE

Perhaps the most significant achievement of the labors of these various groups is found in the area of licensure. In general, a license is a legal document that permits a person to offer to the public his skills and knowledge in a particular jurisdiction, where such practice would otherwise be unlawful without a license. A license to nurse is granted by the appropriate authority to applicants or candidates who have fulfilled certain established requirements. Such a license permits a nurse to practice her profession within the state and gives her the privilege of representing herself as a licensed nurse. A registered nurse has the additional privilege of using the abbreviation "R.N." after her name. The term "certificate" is used for the term "license" in some laws, but the most widely accepted term appears to be "license." The rules for licensing have been created by statutes, and in the application of the law there must be no discrimination, improper pressure or arbitrary action.

The words "for the protection of the public" explain the reason behind the efforts of nursing, both professional and practical, to require licensure for all nurses by the states wherein they practice. The American Nurses' Association has said:

> The primary purpose of a licensing law for the control of the practice of nursing is to protect the health of the people by establishing minimum standards which qualified practitioners must meet.[1]

Exceeding the limits of one's license increases the chance of liability for the nurse and her employer. There was a case in which a practical nurse in a doctor's office administered a polio booster injection to a small child, who suddenly moved; the needle was broken off in the right buttock and, despite surgery, was not located and removed for some months. The parents sued both nurse and doctor for negligence. The trial court exonerated the nurse and doctor but an appellate court reversed the decision, pointing out that under state law only a professional registered nurse may inoculate patients and that the trial judge had failed to so instruct the jury. In addition, the appellate court criticized the lower court for allowing "highly prejudicial" testimony that it was the "custom and practice" in the community for practical nurses to give inoculations, since the practice was contrary to published public policy.[2]

This scope-of-practice problem applies not only to practical nurses, but also to some professional nurses who at times take on the duties of pharmacists and others during the night hours, on weekends, and so forth. Furthermore, the modern clinical specialist, the industrial nurse, the school nurse, the public health nurse and other professional nurse practitioners need to review their work periodically in the light of the scope of practice encompassed by their license.

Permissive Licensure

In contrast to other professions, the law with respect to licensing has been, for the greater part, "permissive." A permissive law applies only to those persons who wish to represent themselves as licensed nurses or to use a title, such as the legal abbreviation, "R.N."

To differentiate mandatory and permissive licensure, the following operational definitions were developed:[3]

> A *mandatory* act requires that anyone who practices nursing according to the definition of the practice that appears in the law must be licensed, the only exceptions being: (1) furnishing nursing assistance in an emergency, (2) practice by student nurses incidental to their course of study, (3) employees of the federal government.*
>
> In a *permissive* act, the titles "registered nurse" and "licensed practical nurse" are protected. The practice of either level of nursing is not prohibited in a permissive act, but an unlicensed person is not entitled to represent himself as an "RN" or an "LPN"‡. In other words, anyone may, whether licensed or not, practice nursing as long as the unlicensed individual does not call himself an RN or an LPN.

Mandatory Licensure

In recent years, there has been what is as yet a limited, though desirable, trend toward mandatory or compulsory licensing in nursing. Mandatory licensing laws control the practice of all who nurse "for hire." Arkansas, Idaho, Louisiana, New Jersey, New York, Rhode Island, Vermont and Hawaii have mandatory licensing laws. Licensing for registered nurses is mandatory according to the boards in Alaska, Arizona, California, Colorado, Connecticut, Illinois, Kansas, Kentucky, Maine, Missouri, Montana, Nevada, New Mexico, Pennsylvania, South Dakota, Washington and Wyoming. Such a mandatory law, though restrictive, does permit relatives or friends to assist others during illness without being penalized by the law. If we really believe that only people with certain basic professional educa-

---

*Nurses in the armed forces or those employed by the Federal Government, often subject to transfer, must hold a current state license but not necessarily from the state to which they are assigned.

‡LPN is interchangeable with LVN, which is preferred in some states, e.g., Texas and California.

tion and experience are qualified to carry out professional nursing functions, then we must make certain that the laws of our state require all those who perform these functions to meet these standards.

Hershey claims that regulating nurses and other health care personnel by mandatory licensing is inefficient and outmoded and suggests an alternative to mandatory licensure:

> Individual licensing of practitioners might be legitimately replaced by investing health services institutions and agencies with the responsibility for regulating the provision of services, within bounds established by the state institutional licensing bodies.[4]

He then goes on to say that the state hospital licensing agency could establish job descriptions for various hospital positions and establish personnel categories in terms of levels or grades. He continues:

> Under the new system, the individual's education and work experience would be considered, and on the basis of this consideration professional nurses could be recognized at any one of three or four grade levels. . . .

This so-called advantage is not new! Professional nurses on the basis of their education and experience are already working at three or four levels.

The purpose of licensure is to protect the public from unskilled and incompetent persons who would practice or offer to practice nursing. To achieve this end, we have worked for years to achieve mandatory rather than permissive licensing statutes. To accept Hershey's proposal now would be to undo years of effort to insure that those who offer nursing service for hire to the public will meet minimum standards of safety and competency. Anyone who can meet the minimum requirements for safety and competency can secure a license to nurse; hence, *if we were to increase the members of nursing personnel through by-passing our mandatory licensing laws, it would be through utilizing those who do not meet the minimum standards for safety and competency*—is this progress? Is it an acceptable alternative to mandatory licensure of nurses?

Furthermore, nursing is a profession. As Lesnik and Anderson have said:

> Historically, one of the characteristics of professions is that they are self-determining; in that certain matters the profession, as the expert group, speaks for itself.[5]

Over the years, nursing has been hampered in its ability to give its best service to the public by individuals and groups on boards of nursing who do not qualify as the most expert in the field of nursing.[6] Now Hershey suggests that the licensing of the individual nurse practitioner (currently based on nation-wide examinations for nurses, written and administered by nurses) be replaced by

> . . . investing health service institutions and agencies with the responsibility for regulating the provision of services, within the bounds established by the state institutional licensing body.

This is clearly robbing nursing of its right to self-determination and control over those who practice.

All violations of the Nursing Practice Act should be reported to the executive secretary of the state board of nurse examiners or similar professional licensing and enforcement groups. The report should include the complete facts of the alleged violation, including the name, time, date and place.[7]

When there has been substantial evidence that a practitioner practiced illegally after his license was revoked, the court has upheld the Licensing Board's refusal to restore his license.[8]

Nurse's Registry

It should be emphasized at the outset that the mere fact that a nurse registers with a registration bureau does not grant her the right to use "R.N." after her name. A registration bureau is really a placement or employment service. The term "nurses' registries" seems to create confusion in the minds of many persons unfamiliar with the practice of nursing and its licensing under the law.

Police Power of the State

Medical and nursing practices are closely allied with and dependent upon each other; though they are similar in their human relationships with the public, only the practice of medicine was early recognized and controlled by law. However, in the last 50 years, nursing has been organized into an occupation with laws regulating the training, education and practices of nurses in the interests of public health, safety and the general welfare. Such laws are based upon what is known as the police power of the state. A good definition of the police power is:

> . . . that inherent sovereignty which the government exercises whenever regulations are demanded by public policy for the benefit of the society at large in order to guard its morals, safety, health, order, and the like, in accordance with the needs of civilization.[9]

DEFINITION OF REGISTERED PROFESSIONAL NURSE

Under this power, laws have been passed prescribing minimum standards of education and training for the practice of different trades, occupations and professions, including nursing. Control over both practice and practitioner protects the public. As Miller stated:

> The purpose of professional licensure is to secure to society the benefits that come from the services of a highly skilled group and on the other hand, to protect society from those, who, being highly skilled, are nevertheless so unprincipled as to misuse their superior knowledge to the disadvantage of people.[10]

The control of nursing practice protects the nurse not only as a member of society, but also in her professional capacity. Licensing is undoubtedly the most important method of legal control and enforcement today.

In 1903, North Carolina adopted the first nursing practice act in the United States. Within 20 years all the states, the District of Columbia and Puerto Rico enacted laws for licensing graduate nurses, usually under the title "Registered Nurse." By 1955, all states had legislation stating in essence that the nurses who wish to practice as full-fledged professional nurses must obtain a license.

Nonstatutory control of professional nursing is accomplished by and through a vigorous, well-organized professional association. As Killough has said:

> It is as legal for the profession to govern itself as it is for any agency of government to control a profession, and if we strive for self-control and view legal control in terms of self control, there will be more contentment within the professions.[11]

While the distinction between medical practice and nursing practice seems clear in the statutes, when specific procedures are considered, the exact line between medical practice and nursing practice is more difficult to determine. Therefore, physicians and nurses need to explore these gray areas of practice together. In New York, for example, a joint committee of the State Medical Society, the State Hospital Association and the New York State Nurses' Association has been established. The three groups agree that the setting and control of standards of practice is the prerogative of each individual profession. They also agree that those problems which arise from the area of joint functioning can be handled best by cooperative effort. As a result of their work, they have issued six joint professional position statements, such as the one on closed-chest cardiac resuscitation and the nurse. The Committee also invites the professional staff of the Nurse Education Office in the State Education Department (which corresponds to the board of nurse examiners in many states) to participate in their meetings. If there is a question about the legal aspects of a procedure, a legal opinion may be obtained from the Department's counsel. When the legality of a nurse's assuming responsibility for a particular procedure is in doubt, an opinion of the state's attorney general may be requested, as was done with respect to the nurse and intravenous therapy.[12]

The California Nurses' Association in cooperation with the California Medical Association and the California Hospital Association similarly have issued joint statements which cover six areas of practice: Intravenous Administration of Fluids, Tuberculin and Other Skin Testing, Noise Control Safety Order, Hypnosis, Closed Chest Cardiac Resuscitation and Administration of Blood.[13]

The Maryland Nurses' Association has an interesting *Report on Protocol on Registered Nurse Responsibilities and Duties as Related to Medical Practice Act*[14] in which they have considered making suggestions relative to 20 medically delegated yet legally questioned procedures nurses have inquired about. The list includes initiation of external cardio-pulmonary resuscitation; administration of investigational drugs; administration of subcutaneous infusions; vena puncture; administration of intravenous (a) fluids, (b) blood, (c) medications, (d) medications added to fluids; removal of inter-cath (indwelling intravenous catheter); deep intratracheal suction; administration of anesthesia during labor; vaginal examination during labor, rectal examination during labor, removal of sutures; suture of minor lacerations; exchange fluids in peritoneal dialysis; performance of tracheotomy; insertion of gastric tubes; "milking" chest tubes to keep them open; interpretation of electro-cardiograms; substitute for pharmacist in his absence; application of pressure bandage to control hemorrhage; and operation of intermittent positive pressure machine.

LICENSED PRACTICAL NURSES

In recent years, another class of licensed nurses, known as licensed practical nurses, has been recognized by the law. All of the states have either permissive or mandatory laws providing for the licensure of practical nurses. These laws vary in some respects in different states. The laws governing the licensure of practical nurses are also based upon the police power and are passed to protect the public from incompetent and unskilled persons who pose as nurses. In states where there is practical nurse licensure, the candidate, upon fulfilling the requirements, is granted the privilege by legal authority to practice and to represent herself as a licensed practical nurse. This is of definite value to the nurse herself, since it indicates that she has met the requirements of the law of the state in which she works.

The National Federation of Licensed Practical Nurses has taken the position that only L.P.N.'s who are graduates of an approved school of practical nursing should be used as charge nurses in extended care facilities, and this has been upheld by the Department of Health, Education and Welfare Report to Congress. This decision was arrived at after careful consideration was given to the problem by numerous consultants in health, education, government and other fields concerned with health care. The report states:

> Their principal concern was to assure, as nearly as standards can assure, a safe level of patient care to [Medicare] beneficiaries. This was considered particularly important in extended care facilities which usually have no house physicians. In these facilities, charge nurses must be prepared to deal with all aspects of patient care, including taking initial action when special problems or medical emergencies arise.[15]

REQUIREMENTS FOR NURSING

Re-registration

Not only do the various jurisdictions require a nurse to obtain a license to practice nursing, but in some states she must also keep her registration up to date by re-registering. The states have boards of nurse examiners which are the legal bodies administering nursing practice acts. The boards of nurse examiners are also called licensing boards, state boards and nursing boards. These boards set up requirements for, and grant state approval to, nursing schools, as well as conduct examinations, issue and renew licenses and certificates of registration, prosecute violators and revoke licenses or certificates. In 1944, the National League for Nursing Education established a national accrediting program for pre-service professional programs in nursing; it is now known as the Accrediting Service of the National League for Nursing, and it has published the *Manual of Accrediting Educational Programs in Nursing*.

Revocation of License

The state board of nurse examiners or some equivalent committee or department is empowered to revoke (or annul) a license for cause. Reasons for revocation may include incompetency, fraud or deceit in securing registration, habitual use of drugs, intemperance, immorality, unprofessional conduct, conviction of a crime involving moral turpitude, aiding or abetting in a criminal abortion, and gross negligence.

In one case, a nurse's license was revoked for unprofessional conduct because she made home visits to patients without either their request or that of their physician, she had diagnosed a patient's condition and advised him that the physician's diagnosis was not correct, she had caused difficulty between patient and physician and she had interfered with family relationships of a patient.[16] On the other hand, the alleged use of profanity has been held insufficient grounds for revoking a professional nurse's license.[17]

When there was substantial evidence that a nurse was guilty of two of the charges filed against her, a New York Court ruled that the revocation of her license was proper, even though she did not appear and defend herself at the hearing before the board, since she admittedly had been notified of the charges against her and of the place, date and time for the hearing in the charges.[18]

Problems of Interstate Licensure

As the licensure of nurses is on a state basis, the laws differ in the various jurisdictions, and thereby give rise to the problem of interstate licensure when nurses move from state to state. In the event that a nurse practitioner who has a license in one state or has completed education and training in one state desires to transfer to a second state to practice her profession, she should write to the board of nurses' examiners in the second state and request information as to requirements, application and examination.

Various factors contribute to the problem of interstate licensure and especially to those who graduated before present evaluating tools were in use.[19] There are a number of practicing nurses whose preparation does not meet the current legal requirements for licensure. Since the last original waiver expired in 1925, and since the last state did not include high school graduation in its law as a requirement for licensure until 1947, it is apparent that a number of middle-aged and older nurses may not have today's entrance requirements for admission to a nursing program. In recent years, common State Board Test Pool examinations have been administered throughout the country, and this is a step in the right direction. However, the same passing score has not been accepted by all states. Again, there is not as yet a commonly accepted quality of nursing program. In the future, the individual's qualifications for licensing may be judged somewhat differently in view of the standards for experimental programs[20] and flexible state education standards in nursing.[21]

Need for uniform laws.   There is a lack of freedom in interstate practice. Obtaining licensure by endorsement (reciprocity) varies from state to state and is not an absolute right. The requirements for licensure in one group of states are the same for candidates by examination and out-of-state applicants, except that an out-of-state nurse does not have to repeat the examination or those parts of it which she passed in the first state. In a second group of states, an out-of-state candidate who fulfills the requirements for license in one state will receive a license by endorsement when the information regarding the original license has been verified with the state which issued it. In a third group of states, an out-of-state applicant may be required to repeat certain items required for licensure, while other items may be accepted after they have been verified with the board which issued the original license.

In some states, an out-of-state applicant may be required to meet present standards. Other states apply standards in effect at the time of graduation or those applicable at the time of original licensing, or the board may have discretionary power in applying its standards to applicants from other states. Evaluation of preparation is easier for nurses who have graduated since the use of common State Board Test Pool examinations throughout the United States.

NURSING PRACTICE ACTS

Although there are nursing practice acts in every state in the country, 11 states have no definition of the practice of nursing in their acts. Nursing practice acts identify areas dealing with the functions of a nurse. Those acts that do define the practice of nursing differ from state to state, but many acts, in defining areas of professional nursing, contain similar provisions.

For example, professional nursing is described in the Louisiana nursing practice act and similarly in the acts of other states as follows:[22]

> 9.3.3 "Practice of Nursing" or "practice of professional nursing" means the performance for compensation of any nursing act in the observation, care and counsel of the ill, injured or infirm, or in the maintenance of health or prevention of illness of others, or in the supervision and teaching of other personnel, and/or the administration of medications and treatments as prescribed by a licensed physician or dentist, requiring substantial specialized judgment and skill and based on knowledge and application of principles of biological, physical and social science, acquired by means of a completed course at an approved school of nursing. The foregoing shall not be deemed to include acts of medical diagnosis or medical prescriptions of therapeutic or corrective nature.
>
> 5. "Registered professional nurse" means any person licensed under this part to engage in the practice of professional nursing as defined in definition No. 3 above.

Nursing Areas and Functions

For further material identifying nursing areas and functions, the reader is referred to the A.N.A. Statement of Functions.[23] In general, the areas of the professional nurse are (1) supervision of a total, comprehensive nursing care plan for the patient, (2) observation, interpretation and evaluation of the patient's symptoms and needs (mental and physical), (3) carrying out the legal orders of physicians for medications and treatments, (4) supervision of auxiliary help (practical nurses, student nurses, other health workers) who give patient care, (5) carrying out nursing procedures and techniques, especially those which require judgment, modification or calculations, based on technical information, (6) giving health guidance and participating in health education, and (7) accurately recording and reporting facts and evaluations of patient care. Lesnik and Anderson have analyzed and discussed at length these nursing areas from the viewpoint of independent and dependent functions.[24]

Importance of Defining Nurse's Work

Lest the reader question the necessity or value of clarifying the functions of a nurse or the boundaries or limits of what is a nurse's work, it is pointed out that such clarification is important to both the nurse and the public (each member of which either is now a patient or is one who may at some future time be a patient of a nurse). To illustrate: If a patient sues a nurse on a charge of malpractice and seeks to recover damages, the patient has to prove that the nurse's negligent act occurred during, or resulted from, her performance of a nursing function, and that she violated the standard of care in her performance of that function. To further illustrate: If a nurse is to avoid such possible charges as practicing medicine unlawfully or malpractice, she must have a clear idea of the duties and functions of a nurse and govern her actions accordingly.

The importance of mandatory licensure was brought out in the case of *Barber v. Reiking.*[25] The mother had taken her 2-year-old boy to a doctor's office for a polio booster shot. The injection was administered by a practical nurse. During the administration of the injection, the boy moved suddenly, and as a result the needle was broken off in his right buttock. Although attempts by surgery and with a magnet were made to remove the needle, it was not recovered until nine months later. In a lawsuit to recover damages for negligence, the language of the licensing law for professional nurses was the controlling factor in the decision, since under it a practical nurse could not legally give an inoculation.

The Court said:

> In accordance with the public policy of this state, one who undertakes to perform the services of a trained or graduate nurse must have the knowledge and skill possessed by a registered nurse. The failure of nurse Reiking to be so licensed raises an inference that she did not possess the required knowledge and skill to administer the inoculation in question. The plaintiff was entitled to have the jury consider this violation of the statute together with the other evidence in the case in determining whether the nurse was negligent.

In discussing the implications of this case, Nathan Hershey correctly observed that nurses who substitute for *de facto* pharmacists by entering the pharmacy to dispense medications at hours when the pharmacist is off duty similarly violate laws pertaining to the practice of pharmacists.[26]

LICENSURE OF PRACTICAL NURSES

In recent years, all states and territories have passed laws controlling practical nursing, and a large number of states have provided for some form of state licensure. There are differences in the laws for the licensure of practical nurses in the various states. Some states have requirements for licensing nursing attendants. Texas licenses trained obstetrical nurses. New Jersey exempts from licensure personnel employed under registered nurse supervision in hospitals, listing specifically:

> ... ward helpers, attendants, technicians, physiotherapists, and medical secretaries.

Schools of Practical Nursing

In a number of states, often in connection with vocational educational programs, a number of fine schools for the education of the practical nurse have developed. The practical nurse should receive a formal course of instruction and supervised clinical experience in a school of nursing which meets the standards approved by the state board of nurses' examiners in a state prescribing licensure. The usual length of the course of instruction is nine months to one year. The National Association of Practical Nurse Education may approve a school of practical nursing, but it acts under no legal authority.

Role of the Practical Nurse

The Statement of Functions of the Licensed Practical Nurse gives this role description:[27]

> The work of the LPN, is an integral part of nursing. The licensed practical nurse gives nursing care under the supervision of the registered professional nurse or physician to patients in simple nursing situations. In more complex situations the licensed practical nurse functions as an assistant to the registered professional nurse.
>
> A simple nursing situation is one that is relatively free of scientific complexity. In a simple nursing situation the clinical state of the patient is relatively stable and the measures of care offered by the physician require abilities based on a comparatively fixed and limited body of scientific facts and can be performed by following a defined procedure step by step. Measures of medical and personal care are not subject to continuously changing and complex modifications because of the clinical and behavioral state of the patient. The nursing that the patient requires is primarily of a physical character and not instructional.

In more complex situations, the licensed practical nurse facilitates patient care by meeting specific nursing requirements of patients as directed, such as preparing equipment, supplies and facilities for patient care, helping the professional nurse to perform nursing measures, and communicating significant observations to the registered professional nurse.

The definitions of practical nursing found in state licensure laws are similar to the one quoted. The definition clarifies the type of nursing a practical nurse will do as well as the leadership she will need. It is necessary for the practical nurse to understand that she must limit her work to the area of authorized practical nursing. She must realize, too, that no physician or registered professional nurse can give her a right to do more than what legally may be done.

Difference Between the Registered Professional Nurse and the Practical Nurse

The essential difference between the registered professional nurse and the practical nurse is that by professional education and training and more refined skills, the registered professional nurse is obliged to evaluate and interpret facts in order to decide necessary action that may be required.

NURSES FROM OTHER COUNTRIES

Professional nurses who are graduates of nursing schools in other countries need help and counseling when they seek licensure in the United States. Many are surprised to learn that they must take an examination for licensure, and some may have to take extra classwork before they can become registered. The American Nurses' Association opposes the active recruitment of nurses from countries which are critically undersupplied. In the case of voluntary immigration of graduate nurses from other countries, the A.N.A. supports their employment on the same basis as their U.S. colleagues, provided they meet the same minimal requirements: (1) adequate educational preparation, (2) state licensure to practice professional nursing, and (3) sufficient command of the English language. A number of alien nurses participate in the Exchange Visitor Program initiated by the Federal Government to improve international understanding through the sharing of knowledge and skills.

IMPORTANCE OF DESIRABLE NURSING LEGISLATION

Progress in any profession is related to the control of practice within that profession. As was pointed out earlier in this chapter, the basis for the licensure of nurses is the police power; i.e., the general welfare of the people makes it necessary in a profession such as nursing that standards be set by the state to protect the public. And if the public is in reality to be protected, the control of nursing practice through licensure needs to be mandatory, rather than permissive, as the majority of laws now are. As nurses and citizens, we should recognize and work for desirable legislation. Moreover, under our form of government, it would seem that each person should receive equal protection.

Need for Uniform Standards of Nursing

At present, protection varies with the variety of standards for the practice of nursing in the different states. The requirements for the practice of nursing remain under the state's jurisdiction, but standards in nursing, as in other professions, ought to be developed by the profession on a national basis. The activities of the subcommittees of the A.N.A. Special Committee on State Boards of Nursing concerning more flexible standards, as well as the Accrediting Service of the National League for Nursing, are an illustration of the activities and studies needed.

Nurses' Interest in Legislation

Nurses must be interested in laws and study their effect on the profession. In the different states, the administration of the law is the work of the board of nurse examiners or an equivalent group, and therefore board members are public servants. The influence of such an administrative agency may be appreciable, and if the intent of nursing practice laws, namely, to provide for the public welfare, is to be achieved, it would seem that the criteria for selecting such board members should be their competence, expertness and knowledge in the field of nursing. Nurses professionally organized must thoughtfully look to the intent of the law and how best to achieve that intent. The preceding examples of the law and its relation to the nurse are by no means an inclusive list of problems or problem areas, nor are they necessarily the greatest or most urgent problems, but rather they illustrate the point that nurses need to know and be concerned with the law, especially in relation to their calling.

VALUE OF NURSING PUBLICATIONS AND PROFESSIONAL NURSING ORGANIZATIONS

Laws are being modified continually; after a nurse has left school perhaps the best way for her to keep up with current changes that may affect her is through the the medium of the monthly nursing publications which serve the profession. One of the chief objectives of the professional nursing organizations is to try to secure adequate nursing legislation in all states. Reports and discussions of such matters in her periodicals keep the nurse up-to-date on the legal aspects of her profession.

REFERENCES

1. Principles of Legislation Relating to Nursing Practice. American Nurses' Association, New York. Rev. January, 1958
2. Barber v. Reiking, 411 P.2d 861 (Wash., 1966). See *The Physicians Legal Brief* (Schering) 8 (7) 2, Sept., 1966 and Hershey, Nathan: A Court's View of Mandatory Licensure. *Am. J. Nursing,* 66:2461-2, Nov. 1966
3. Report of AMA Committee on Nursing Mandatory vs. Permissive Licensure for Nurses. *J.A.M.A.,* 195:202-3, Feb. 7, 1966. Prepared by Florence M. Alexander, Ph.D., R.N., formerly director of AMA Department of Nursing
4. Hershey, Nathan: An Alternative to Mandatory Licensure of Health Professionals. *Hosp. Progr.,* 50:71-4, March, 1969
5. Lesnik, Milton J., and Anderson, Bernice E.: Nursing Practice and the Law. Philadelphia, Lippincott, 1955, p. 87
6. *Idem.*
7. Violations of Law Should be Reported. *Wash. State J. Nurs.,* 36:10, Sept., 1964
8. Illinois Appellate Court Upholds Dental Board's Refusal to Restore Plaintiff's Dental License. *Am. Dental Assn. J.,* 77:34, July, 1968
9. Miami County v. Dayton, 92 Ohio St. 215, 110 N.E. 726 (1915)
10. Miller, Justin: The Philosophy of Professional Licensure. Proceedings of the Annual Congress on Medical Education, Licensure and Hospitals, Chicago, February 12-13, 1934
11. Killough, Robert C.: Legal Control of Professional Practice. (Speech delivered at the conference for State Boards of Nursing, May, 1959)
12. Schmidt, Mildred S.: Legal Considerations in Nursing. New York State Nurse, 40:12-16, Nov., 1968
13. Papers Fix Joint Responsibility. *The CNA Bulletin,* 61:1, Nov., 1965
14. MNA Statement on "Report on Protocol on Registered Nurse Responsibilities and Duties as Related to Medical Practice Act," Maryland Nursing News, 34:10-12, Fall, 1965. Also available from the Maryland Nurses' Association: Statement on Closed Chest Cardiac Resuscitation and Artificial Respiration by the Registered Professional Nurse; Statement on Intravenous Administration of Fluids, Blood, Medications by Professional Registered Nurses Practicing in Maryland; Statement on Nurses' Responsibilities in Dispensing Drugs During the Absence of a Pharmacist; Joint Statement Regarding the Professional Relationships of the Practicing Members of the Maryland Nurses Association and the American Physical Therapy Association of Maryland; and Joint Statement of the Role of the Registered Nurse in the Care of the Patients with Cardiovascular Diseases in Coronary Care or Intensive Care Units
15. NFLPN Position on Charge Nurses in Extended Care Facilities Upheld by Department of Health, Education and Welfare Report to Congress. *Bedside Nurse,* 2:45-46, March-Apr., 1969
16. Stefanik v. Nursing Educational Committee, 37 A 2d 661 (R.I., 1944)
17. Colorado State Board of Nurse Examiners v. Hahn, 129 Col. 195, 268 P 2d 401 (1954)
18. Lanaro v. Allen, 259 N.Y.S. 2d 366 (N.Y., 1965)
19. Anderson, Bernice E.: The Facilitation of Interstate Movement of Registered Nurses. Philadelphia, Lippincott, 1950; The Problem of Interstate Licensure. *Am. J. Nursing,* 52:587-9, 1952
20. Anderson, Bernice E.: State Board Requirements and Experimental Programs. *Am. J. Nursing,* 54:67-8, 1954

21. Guide for Use of State Boards in Developing Standards for Accrediting Pre-Service Education Programs Preparing Professional Nurses. ANA Special Committee of State Boards of Nursing. New York, American Nurses' Association, 1959

22. Louisiana Revised Statutes of 1950, Title 37, Ch. II, Part I as amended by Act 166, July 27, 1966, comprising Sections 911 through 939

23. A.N.A. Statement of Functions. *Am. J. Nursing*, 54:868-71, 992-6, 1130, 1954

24. Lesnik, Milton J., and Anderson, Bernice E.: Nursing Practice and the Law. Philadelphia, Lippincott, 1955, p. 258 ff. and p. 380 ff.

25. 68 W2 139, 411 P. 2d 861 (1966)

26. Hershey, Nathan: A Court's View of Mandatory Licensure. *Am. J. Nursing*, 66:2461-2, Nov., 1966. See also Schering, *The Physician's Legal Brief.* 8 (7) 2, Sept., 1966

27. Statement of Functions of the Licensed Practical Nurse, *Am. J. Nursing*, 64:93, Mar., 1964.

Chapter Three

Contracts for Nursing

When a nurse enters the active practice of her profession, she will become involved in contracts of one type or another. It is therefore necessary for her to have at least basic information on contracts and agreements. Moreover, it is of value to know that at law there is also a remedy for one party or the other for the breaking of a legal contract. The nurse should know her rights and, on the other hand, the rights of the other party, so that she may avoid trouble.

DEFINITION OF CONTRACTS

A contract has been defined as a promise, or a set of promises, the performance of which the law recognizes as a duty, and when that duty is not performed, the law provides a remedy.[1]

REQUIREMENTS OF CONTRACTS

Every contract, to be enforceable at law, must contain (1) the real consent of the parties (persons), (2) a valid consideration (something of value), (3) a lawful object (purpose), (4) competent parties (persons with a legal capacity to make a contract), and (5) the form required by law. Under the law of contracts there is a remedy for a breach of contract so that the person who suffers from a broken contract may gain recompense of some sort.

Although every contract is an agreement between two or more parties, not every agreement is a contract. For instance, one may agree to play a musical instrument at a party as a favor for a friend, or a person who has not attended church in years may agree to meet another and to attend a church service with him. If either person to such an agreement, for any reason, failed to do what he had agreed to do, it would not be considered a binding agreement for which he would be liable to penalty under the law. In general, moral agreements, agreements of conscience or agreements involving social obligations are not classified as contracts.

Offer and Acceptance

In any contract there must be an offer and an acceptance. For example, Miss A offers to do or refrain from doing something for Miss B, and Miss B accepts the offer of Miss A. An offer must be definite, it must be communicated by words or actions, and it may be withdrawn before it is accepted. If Hospital C telephones Mr. Smith that it has a bed ready for him today, Mr. Smith's coming to Hospital C today is acceptance. Since a person has the right to choose those with whom he will do business, an acceptance of an offer is good only if it comes from the person to whom the offer was made. Another rule provides that acceptance must be unconditional and in accord with the contract's terms as to price, amount, time of delivery, etc.

The person making the offer can terminate it at any time. It is effective when communication of such termination is received by the person to whom the offer was made. If the person who makes the offer accepts a payment in return for agreeing not to revoke the offer for a certain period of time, the offer is thereby converted into an option. The law treats the option as a binding contract that cannot be terminated during the time period.

Consideration

In addition to the elements of an offer and an acceptance, there must also be "consideration" for the contract. As an example, Mr. Jones, a private patient, enters Hospital C. Care given Mr. Jones by the hospital is "consideration" for his promise to pay proper charges.

As long as the consideration constitutes a bargained-for exchange, its fairness is irrelevant.

In some states, action by a party receiving a gratuitous promise, in reliance on that promise, can be a legally sufficient consideration to make the promise enforceable as a contract. For example, in a recent New York case, during a construction fund-raising campaign to build a hospital, the defendant doctor was asked to pledge a sum of money and he did so. The doctor paid $500 toward his pledge during the next four years. Then the hospital brought suit when he refused to pay the balance of his pledge. The appellate court gave judgment to the hospital for the balance due on its pledge. The court said:

> It is the well established law of this State that charitable subscriptions (pledges) are enforceable on the ground that they constitute an offer of a unilateral contract which, when accepted by the charity by incurring liability and reliance thereon, becomes a binding obligation.[2]

The new hospital was built, so the hospital had fulfilled its obligation under the pledge.

KINDS OF CONTRACTS

There are formal contracts and simple or parol (verbal) contracts, as well as implied contracts and express contracts.

Formal Contracts

A *formal* contract is one required by law to be in writing. As an example, each state has its Statute of Frauds, which requires written contracts in specified cases in order to prevent fraudulent practices. Mortgages, deeds and similarly important papers are often printed on a paper on which a seal or the use of the word "seal" shows that it is a contract under seal, another kind of formal contract.

Simple Contracts

Other contracts, whether written or oral, are called simple or parol contracts.

Express Contracts

An express contract is one in which the conditions and terms of the contract are given orally or in writing by the parties. For example, Hospital C offers Miss Jones, in writing, a position as a staff nurse at a salary of $640 per month for a five-day week consisting of 40 hours, and Miss Jones accepts the offer in writing. Here the terms are expressed. It should be pointed out that a contract is not necessarily written.

Implied Contracts

On the other hand, suppose Miss Jones goes to Dr. Smith's office and Dr. Smith gives Miss Jones professional services which she accepts. This is an implied contract. Perhaps the greater number of contracts which we encounter in daily living are implied. The sale and purchase of many commodities is an example of a simple implied contract. We go to a store that has food, another store that has clothing, or another that has various supplies, all for sale. The store offers the various items for sale at a price. We expect to and do pay the price asked, and we obtain the article. Our contract is completed.

Silent contracts. The implied contract may also be referred to as a silent contract. The consent is silent. For example, Hospital C places all the features of an employment contract before Miss Jones, and after reading it Miss Jones enters on duty. The performance of the act is acceptance. However, one person, by including a statement such as "Unless I hear to the contrary, I will consider my offer accepted by you," cannot make a second person accept the offer through keeping quiet. In other words, silence, unless there is a duty from the circumstances to speak, is not an acceptance of an offer.

Oral contracts are the most common, and many employment contracts fall into this category. The employer and the employee talk things over and come to an agreement as to what services shall be performed for a specified compensation. The terms and payments may be simple or complicated, but they are binding on both parties.

Courts consistently hold that oral contracts for a year or more are void. Parker cites a recent decision regarding an oral contract under which a physician was employed by hospital officials for one year at a salary of $28,000.[3] Following a disagreement at the end of six months, the hospital officials discharged the physician after paying him only $12,000. The hospital was held not liable in damages for breaching the oral contract, since a contract for one year was void and unenforceable.

APPLICATION OF BASIC FACTS OF CONTRACTS TO NURSES AND NURSING SERVICE

It has been shown that a contract is an agreement between two or more persons for a consideration. In all contracts, there is mutual consent or a willingness by both parties that the acts will be performed.

Nurses' Contracts

When a nurse enters into a professional employment agreement, it is desirable and it is recommended that it be executed in writing, especially if it is anticipated that it will exist for a period of more than one year. Nevertheless, many nurses err in assuming that since they have no written contract, they have no binding legal commitment. From a legal point of view, there is, based on mutual understanding and followed by performance of professional services and payment for the same, a personal service contract that is binding. The nurse has the duty to perform her nursing assignment in accordance with the standards of professional nursing practice as defined by the profession and in the nursing practice act of the state. The employer has the duty to provide not only a safe place to work and safe equipment with which to work, but also properly trained and qualified co-workers.[4]

In the case of a private duty nurse's contract, the nurse agrees to serve a patient and the patient agrees to pay the nurse for the service. Possibly the patient has a relative or friend acting for him as his agent, or two persons agree to pay a nurse for the services rendered to the patient. Likewise, a nurse may have an agent acting for her. Agreements involving agents will be discussed in subsequent paragraphs.

Definite commitments. Nurses' contracts should be made as definite as possible concerning the various terms in the offer and acceptance. Otherwise, the law may be called upon to interpret or clarify the uncertainties.

HOURS AND SALARY. If one of the points, such as the amount of daily wage, is indefinite rather than specific, then the law determines such according to what is "reasonable." In a given case, what is reasonable depends upon local custom in such a situation. For instance, if Town A engages a nurse, Miss Jones, as a public health nurse at an annual salary equivalent to that paid by a neighboring community, the fixed terms and usage can be readily ascertained.

For a private duty nurse, the hours and the pay are usually inferred. In the absence of an express statement, compensation is at the rate prevailing in the locality.

LENGTH OF CONTRACT. Again, unless the patient ends the contract earlier, or unless there is a stipulation providing otherwise, the time a contract runs with a private duty nurse generally coincides with the duration of the patient's need or illness. It is the usual assumption that the patient or someone acting for him understands that the nursing service contract of the private duty nurse is on a day-to-day basis and that the nurse will serve as long as the patient desires her services. The prevailing custom is that the patient has the right to terminate the private duty nurse's services at any time, but the nurse does not enjoy the same right.

When a hospital, institution or agency enters into a valid employment contract with a nurse or doctor for a specified time, then the party who willfully breaches such contract may be held liable in damages. Thus in U.S. v. Averick the Veterans Administration sued a doctor for breach of a contract and recovered $20,616 damages.[5] Under the terms of the contract, the physician was to receive medical training in pathology while employed full-time as a physician, with a provision that he was to remain in the employ of the V.A. for a length of time equal to the residency period after its completion. In the event that the physician failed to complete the agreed period of service after his residency, the contract provided for liquidated damages of $492 per month for each month owed but not worked. When the doctor resigned from the V.A. after four years of training, suit was brought and he was held liable for breach of contract. Similarly, in a case in which an employee was discharged without good cause at the end of six months, whereas he had a written contract of employment for one year at $200 per month, the employer had to pay six months' salary as damages.[6]

DAYS OFF-DUTY. At the negotiation of the contract, and before entering upon duty, the private duty nurse has the right to limit the length of her services on the case, for example, to a week, two weeks, or a month, or she may well desire to incorporate specific provisions for "relief" or days off-duty. For example, if a patient, Mr. Brown, makes a contract with a nurse, Miss Jones, for nursing care, Miss Jones cannot as a matter of right, in the absence of a specific provision, take a day off and send another nurse, Miss Smith, as a substitute.

LOCAL CUSTOM. As for the length of time which other contracts for nursing services run, in the absence of a definite statement, local custom is an important factor in the determination. The Dakotas, California and Montana have applicable statutes on this subject. There is also some authority found in court decisions to the effect that in contracts for services, the period such a contract runs in any event is not less than the salary specified; i.e., so much per week or month may be taken to indicate a hiring for that period. When nurses are employed by hospitals, agencies and institutions, employment by the month is often assumed in the absence of a specific provision or local custom.

As for the wages or salary to be paid for the various nursing services, the inclusion of definite terms in contracts is desirable. In the absence of a provision for a specific amount, the nurse's compensation depends on what is reasonable. The amount that is reasonable depends upon what others in the same area are usually receiving for comparable services. It should be noted that when such a question arises, the nurse who wants to collect for the services performed would have the burden of verifying what is a "reasonable" compensation.

Sometimes disputes arise as to whether an oral contract for a nurse's services should have been put in writing. In the case of *Cox v. Baltimore,* a nurse made an oral contract to work at $100.00 a week for the patient for life, and such a contract was held to be valid.[7]

Details of duties and functions. Sometimes disputes arise as to what does constitute the "services" of a nurse. Details of duties and functions may vary from area to area, not only for private duty nurses and general duty nurses, but also with regard to nursing school administrators, nurse consultants, teachers of nursing, public health nurses, nurse directors of mining services and other industrial nurses, nurse supervisors, practical nurses, and others in the field. Again, local custom has some bearing on what is expected of a nurse in a given position. As guides, the reader is referred to the American Nurses' Association Statement of Functions[8] for information on registered professional nurses and to the Practical Nursing Curriculum[9] for duties and functions of the practical nurse.

Explanation of Offer and Acceptance

At times a nurse's contract or attempt to contract presents a problem because "offer" and "acceptance" are not fully understood. When an offer is made, it is well to realize that it may be withdrawn before it is accepted. For example, if Mr. Brown sends an offer to Miss Jones and then changes his mind before she has accepted the offer, this is his privilege and he incurs no penalty.

Reasonable period for acceptance. Moreover, when an offer is made, it is not indefinitely open for acceptance. Either the offer itself states that it must be accepted within a given period, or, if no time is set, such an offer would be considered open for a "reasonable period." What constitutes a "reasonable period" depends upon the circumstances of each case. An offer may be rejected, and it is therefore no longer open for acceptance.

Means used to accept offer. A point of difference as to whether or not an offer has been accepted might arise if a different means is used to accept the offer than was used in making the offer. For instance, if an offer is made in a letter written by some person or agency to a nurse, the law provides that the person making the offer authorize the person receiving the offer to use the same means in sending his acceptance, i.e., by letter through the mail. Under this arrangement, the law considers that acceptance has been made and that the contract is completed when the person receiving the offer replies by the same means, dropping his letter of acceptance (properly addressed and stamped) in the mail box. On the other hand, if a person mails an offer to a nurse and the nurse replies by wire, the contract is complete only when the person who made the offer receives the wire of acceptance, and not when the nurse sent the telegram. Though to a nurse this may seem like splitting hairs, it is the law of contracts; and since it might be important to the nurse in some cases, she should consider carefully the means by which she replies to an offer.

Illegal Contracts

The question of legality of a contract may arise, for a court will not enforce an illegal contract. The use of fraud (deception, trickery), undue (unlawful) influence or duress (coercion) in securing a contract will make it illegal. An agreement providing for a higher rate of interest than is allowed by law, or one amounting to undertaking to commit a crime is illegal, as is also any attempt to obstruct justice. Of importance to nurses is the fact that in certain states the law requires a nurse to be licensed, and if a nurse in such states does not obtain a license, then any contract for nursing service that she makes may be held illegal.* Furthermore, if a nurse in making a contract claims to be an R.N. or licensed P.N., and in fact is not, the contract is not enforceable even in a state with permissive licensure. In such instances, if the nurse does give nursing service to a patient and the patient does not pay her, the nurse may be unable to recover any money for her services, if the illegality of the contract is set up as a defense.

There are times when two or more persons may undertake a joint responsibility to pay for care of a patient. For example, two sons employ and agree to pay for a nurse to care for their father or mother. This is an enforceable agreement often referred to as a contract for the benefit of a third person.

Definition of Agent and Principal

An agent is a person designated by another, called the principal, to do, perform or act in an authorized manner in the name of the principal, but always subject to the control or wishes of the principal.[10] When he so acts, the agent binds the principal. It should be noted that one cannot delegate to an agent the performance of an agreement involving personal services.†

A patient in need of nursing service may ask a physician to obtain a nurse. When the physician does so, he is acting as the patient's agent. The patient as the principal is bound by the contract. In another instance, the nurse may act as an agent. For example, she is requested by a patient to obtain a nurse for him, and she does so. The patient is bound to pay the nurse who has been secured for him.

Nurses' registries. Sometimes an agent, such as a nurses' registry, supplies the nurse requested by the patient. There are different kinds of registries with varying authority and status, and the distinctions should be noted by the nurse.

OFFICIAL REGISTRY FOR NURSES. For example, there is the official registry for nurses, which is usually supported to a greater or lesser extent by charges and fees of the nurses it lists. When a patient or someone acting for him requests such registry to obtain a nurse for him and the registry does so, it is usually regarded as the agent of the patient. Though the nurse pays the official registry for having em-

---

*See Chapter II for an explanation of mandatory versus permissive licensure.

†See Section 17c of Reference 4; also the comment on Sections 400, 401, 406 and 409, which states the consequences which may follow an improper delegation.

ployment opportunities brought to her attention, customarily she does not give it power to act in her name as her agent.

HOSPITAL REGISTRY. Similarly, hospital registries, whether separate or a part of the hospital service, are not designated by nurses as agents acting for such nurses, but rather become the agent of the patient when asked to supply a nurse.

NURSES' REGISTRY OPERATED FOR PROFIT. When a nurses' registry is operated for profit, customarily there is a contract designating such registry as the agent of either nurse or patient, or both, and specifying the person obligated to pay the registry.

GRATUITOUS AGENCY. In the gratuitous agency, if there is a failure on the part of the agent to secure employment for a nurse, it cannot be considered a breach of contract for which there is a remedy, because there was no contract.

Consideration, as noted, is an essential element of a contract, but consideration is not an essential element in setting up an agency relationship. It should be noted that a contract made by an agent who acts gratuitously is just as binding on the principal as one made by an agent who receives recompense therefor.

Agent's responsibility for negligent acts. If Agent A, while acting for Principal B, injures a third person, Miss Jones, through some negligent act, (1) Agent A himself can be sued for money damages by the third person, Miss Jones, and (2) Principal B, for whom Agent A acted, can also be sued for money damages.

Questions concerning whether or not a person is acting as an agent, and for whom the agent is acting, can be important in situations involving nurses. For example, a patient asked a student nurse to inquire of his doctor whether he might go home, and the student nurse said she would, but negligently failed to do so. In this case the patient went home after receiving his bill and later found that he had a fractured leg. An action by the patient to recover damages proved unsuccessful because the court held that the hospital could not be charged with the student nurse's negligence, since she was acting as the patient's agent and not the agent of the hospital.[11]

If a nurse acts as agent, she is responsible for her own negligent acts, regardless of whether she acts gratuitously or for pay. Similarly, a nurses' registry is responsible for negligent acts due to a failure to do what can reasonably be expected of such registries. For example, Mr. Brown requested Registry A to send him a nurse, and Registry A sent a nurse who was listed with it. An ordinary reasonable check on the character and credentials usually made by registries would have shown this person to be an alcoholic, but Registry A failed to check. Several days later, Mr. Brown was injured by a wrong medication given by the nurse while she was working under the influence of alcohol. Mr. Brown could bring suit against Registry A as well as against the nurse to recover damages for injury caused by negligence.

EXCEPTION FOR CHARITABLE INSTITUTIONS. One exception to the above illustration should be noted. If Registry A is a part of a charitable institution, then in states where charitable institutions cannot be sued for negligence, Registry A could not be sued for negligence. Of course, this does not prevent the patient, Mr. Brown, from suing the nurse, but he may have great difficulty in collecting any judgment for damages.

Wife as agent of husband. In dealing with agencies, an agency implied by the law must be considered. In some situations, the law implies an agency through which one person may bind a second person to a contract, although the matter has not been considered by the latter. For example, in case of a husband and wife living together, the wife usually buys what they need on her husband's credit account. The wife is his agent under these circumstances. If the husband becomes ill or injured and is a patient in a hospital, the wife continues as his agent, and the law would in all likelihood recognize her authority to engage a nurse needed for his care. The husband, as principal, is bound by the contract to compensate such a nurse. If the wife were the patient, the husband ordinarily is responsible for necessary services (including nursing service) to his wife. In the latter case, it is the husband's legal duty while they are living together to provide for his wife.

The situation is different if the husband and wife are living apart. She may have left him without cause, prompting the husband to give notice that he is no longer responsible for her purchases. In such cases, the husband will not have to pay the wife's bill.

HUSBAND LIABLE FOR NECESSARIES OF WIFE AND MINOR CHILDREN. The private duty nurse may well be interested in ascertaining who is liable for payment of her wages. In all jurisdictions, by law a husband must supply his wife with necessities. If a husband does not supply necessities, a wife as agent for the husband may buy the necessities even without his consent.[12] Assume in such a case that a wife, as agent for her husband, who does not furnish her nursing care, nevertheless contracts with a nurse to secure "necessary" nursing care for herself. How may the nurse collect her fees? To do so, the nurse would have to prove that the husband was at fault in not supplying nursing care for his wife; or if the husband and wife live apart, the nurse must establish that the husband was to blame.

Again, if a husband is obliged to support a minor child, it would seem that a wife acting under an implied agency could contract with a nurse to give "necessary" nursing service to the child and bind the husband to the contract.[13] In such a case, in the event that a nurse deals with a wife and intends to contract only with the wife and not the husband, then only the wife is responsible.

Nursing service a necessity. In general, medical, nursing and hospital services are necessities. Parents are legally responsible in the majority of states for providing necessities to their minor children. However, when parents give up control and supervision of a minor and he keeps his own wages, he may be regarded as "emancipated" (freed) even though he continues to live at home. In such a case, a father is not liable for services given the child. Also, a nurse could not charge the parents for services given a married minor child, since marriage emancipates or releases the child from parental responsibility.

Real Consent

It has been shown that, to have a contract, there must be two or more persons, an offer, an acceptance and a consideration. In addition, to have a legally enforceable contract, it is often said that there must be real consent, i.e., a "meeting of the minds," revealing the lack of misrepresentation or fraud of real significance. To be able to make valid contracts, persons must have legal capacity.

Disability to make binding contracts. Certain groups of persons are under a disability to make binding contracts, but legal capability is presumed unless one of the following grounds exists: mental incompetence, marital disqualification, infancy, intoxication or drug addiction to a degree precluding legal transactions.

Mental incompetence. Persons to a contract must be mentally competent, i.e., not suffering from a mental disease or defect. Determining whether a person is mentally competent either for medical or for legal purposes is a thorny and difficult matter, as many nurses realize from some training or duty in psychiatric hospitals. The persons must be capable of understanding the conditions and necessary or natural result of the contract.

Legal insanity. Legal insanity is often determined by the so-called right and wrong test, based on the rule in *McNaghten's Case*.[14, 15]

> A man is sane when he knows that nature and quality of his acts and knows that they are wrong.

In a recent decision in the District of Columbia, the court, after a review of existing tests based on the accused's knowledge of the difference between right and wrong as supplemented by the irresistible impulse test, rejected the same as the only criteria for determining criminal responsibility. The court substituted a rule that an accused is not criminally responsible if his wrongful act is the product of mental disease or mental defect.[16] As a basis for avoiding a contract, insanity does not mean:

> ... a total deprivation of reason, but an inability from defect of perception, memory and judgment to do the act in question or to understand its natural consequences.[17]

Also, it must appear that the insanity existed at the time of the particular contract, i.e., that because of the diseased condition of his mind, the person made a contract which he would not have made had he been rational.[18]

As generally used in the popular sense, insanity refers to varying degrees of unsoundness of mind, and people realize that sometimes there is a close line between sanity and insanity. Moreover, insanity may be a temporary condition, and a person may have a lucid interval when he is sane enough to be considered as being in a normal state. This makes the matter much more difficult to determine, especially when a person has not been declared insane by a court, since he may make a contract during such an interval, and the contract is valid.

Generally, contracts made by an insane person are voidable; that is, when and if the insane person regains his sanity, he may affirm or repudiate the contract. However, the other party to the contract cannot use such insanity as an excuse to avoid the contract.

When there is a want of sufficient mental capacity to transact ordinary business and to take care of and manage property, the law will authorize the appointment of a guardian for the patient.[19] If a person is incompetent, but has not been declared so judicially, statutes in the different states provide that an action for the appointment of a guardian may be brought by his next friend, who is either a volunteer or one appointed by the court. After a person has been declared incompetent or insane at law, any contracts he makes are void; but his guardian has legal authority to act in his place. An insane or incompetent person is liable for necessities for himself, his wife and his minor children. Medical service including nursing, has been held to be necessity.[20] In a case decided 80 years ago, the court held that a husband may not withhold necessary medical assistance for his wife by not giving consent to an operation.[21]

Marital disqualification. According to the common law (the law prior to passage of a statute), husband and wife were "one"; hence, during the husband's lifetime (unless he were imprisoned for life or deserted her) a married woman had no legal capacity to make a contract, although a single woman had such capacity. At common law, if a married woman wished to make any sort of contract, even if it concerned land and movable articles that she had before marriage or inherited after marriage, she needed the consent of her husband.

The disability of married women has been generally overcome by statutes in each state as society and the economic aspects of life have changed in form and tempo. Under the Married Women's Acts, a married woman can own property in her own name and can, through an express contract, make herself personally liable for necessities supplied to her and her family. However, the nurse should remember that unless the married woman binds herself personally for nursing services rendered to her, she is not liable for the services.

Infancy. At common law, a contract made by a minor was voidable, and a person retained the power to disaffirm a contract until the day before reaching 21 years of age. Today, a person under the age of 21 years is still regarded as an infant unless the age limit has been changed by statute in a particular jurisdiction.

A man or woman attains full capacity to contract upon marriage in Louisiana, Iowa, Kansas and Utah. In addition, in the following states a woman attains full capacity to contract upon marriage: Maryland, Alabama, Texas, Nebraska, California, Oregon and Washington. In the states of Maryland, Arkansas, Illinois, Minnesota, North Dakota, South Dakota, Montana, Utah, Nevada, Idaho and Oregon a woman attains full capacity at 18 years.[21]

BIRTH CONTROL PILL FOR MINORS. Nurses and physicians frequently encounter in clinics or the doctor's office an unmarried teenage girl who seeks birth control pills to protect her against pregnancy. She is not accompanied by her parent nor does she wish the parent to be contacted for a consent for the requested treatment; hence two questions arise: (1) is the teenage girl's own consent legally sufficient for treatment? and (2) should this request for treatment be brought to the parent's attention?[22]

Whether or not the teenage girl can lawfully consent to treatment generally depends upon whether she is an emancipated minor or not. Except in a state that has a statute specifying another age, a person under the age of 21 years is considered a minor or not of age. In a limited number of states, a child may petition the courts to remove the disability of infancy. In other states, the minor may be emancipated if the parents relinquish their responsibility to control and care for the minor, as well as their rights to his services and earnings. When a minor marries, the parents' control ceases. Accordingly, unless the teenage girl is emancipated, the consent of her parents or guardian is needed before treatment. Therefore, the physician should endeavor to persuade the girl to bring her parent in to discuss the requested treatment, or, in lieu thereof, to allow the physician to seek the parent's consent for treatment. Where the teenage girl is unwilling to have the physician contact her parents for consent to treat her, he still may lawfully disclose such a request for treatment to them in the typical situation. Whether in fact the physician does disclose to parents the request for a prescription for birth control pills is more a question of discretion than law.

Definition of voidable contract. Contracts made with minors are voidable, but not void. This statement needs explanation, since it may seem contradictory. A voidable contract is one that may be valid in every way except that one of the persons has the option of rejecting it. Such a power is given to the minor who makes a contract. For example, if John Brown, a 19-year-old movie star, contracts with Miss Jones, a nurse, to pay for nursing service for his 16-year-old sister,

Sue Brown, before John Brown becomes 21 years old, he may pay the charges or reject the contract. Obviously, the benefits of nursing service are a consideration that cannot be returned in case he rejects the contract.

Definition of void contract. A void contract is one prohibited by law or public policy that creates no rights. For example, a contract made by a person legally declared insane is void.

A minor's contract is voidable until he decides to affirm (give positive approval) or avoid it. According to common law, in a contract for real estate, the minor had to wait until he was 21 years old to affirm or avoid the contract. If the contract concerned personal property (any item of movable or immovable property except real estate or things which are a part of it), the minor could reject it at any time, even prior to attaining his legal age. The rejection could be verbal (oral) or in writing, or it could be implied from his conduct. Upon rejecting the contract, if the minor has received any of the consideration for the contract, he must return it. However, in general, if the minor has used, lost or destroyed what he received as consideration, he still may reject the contract. According to decided cases, in some states, an infant at any age, and according to some statutes a minor over 18 years, cannot reject a contract unless he returns what he has received.[23]

Under statutes today, some contracts made by a minor, such as marriage, enlistment in the armed forces, or for necessities to be supplied to him, are obligatory or binding. Among other things, necessities have been held to include medical service.[24] What is a necessity varies somewhat with the person's economic and social status.

The minor is liable only for the reasonable value of necessities supplied to him. For example, when a minor has received necessities, it should be noted that while the "reasonable value" may not exceed the contract price, neither is a "reasonable value" necessarily the contract price. A nurse should be aware of the legal aspects and be careful when making contracts with minors. She should remember that in such a contract, if the minor wants to reject it, the contract is open to investigation and determination by law regarding the necessity of her services and the reasonableness of their value, and that the burden of proving both these facts is on her.

CONCLUSIONS

Restatement of Requirements for Valid Contract

An agreement, to be an enforceable contract, includes the real consent of the persons, valid consideration, a lawful object, competent parties and the form required by law. In general, the rule is that, to

40 LAW EVERY NURSE SHOULD KNOW

be "competent parties," the persons must be capable of understanding the meaning and consequences of their acts. If persons do not have the mental capacity (irrespective of the cause) to understand the statements in the agreement, then such contract is voidable, or when the person has been declared legally incompetent, the contract is void. In addition to insanity, the lack of mental capacity may arise from different causes: the influence of liquor or drugs, old age, senility, and a variety of diseases and disabilities which make a person unable to conduct the ordinary affairs of his life. Whether or not an intoxicated person can make a valid contract depends in part on the degree of intoxication: a slight intoxication possibly might not affect his mental capability, whereas an intoxicated person might be, on the other hand, as lacking in contractual capacity as a person temporarily insane. Statutes in different states make provision for having habitual drunkards as well as other persons incapacitated by various disabilities declared legally incompetent, and a guardian appointed for them. A contract made by any person declared legally incompetent is void; his guardian, however, has authority to act for him.

Contracts for necessities to be supplied to such incompetent parties, their wives and minor children are binding. Nursing services have been held "necessities."[25] However, the nurse who attempts to recover on such contracts must prove that her services were necessary and that the charges cover only "reasonable" compensation.

REFERENCES

1. Cox v. Baltimore & O.S.W.R. Co., 180 Ind. 495, 103 N.E. 337 (1913)
2. Cohoes Memorial Hospital v. Mossey, 266 N.Y.S. 501 (1966)
3. Parker, Leo T.: Review of Hospital Lawsuits. *Hosp. Topics,* 43:69, 86, Jan., 1965, and 43:78, Aug., 1965
4. Regan, William A.: Contract for Nursing Service. *Regan Report on Nursing Law,* 4 (8) 1, Jan., 1965
5. United States v. Averick, 249 F. Supp. 237 (1965)
6. Cavalier v. Weinstein, 80 A. 2d 918 (1951)
7. Cox v. Baltimore & O.S.W.R. Co., 180 Ind. 495, 103 N.E. 337 (1913)
8. American Nurses' Association: Statement of Functions. Am. J. Nursing, 54:868-71, 994-6, 1130, 1954
9. Available from Wisconsin Association of Practical Nurses, 1500 Orchard St., Racine, Wis.; Statement of Functions of the Licensed Practical Nurse. *Am. J. Nursing,* 64:93, Mar., 1964
10. *Restatement, Agency,* 1933, § 17c.
11. Bowdich v. French Broad Hospital, 201 N.C. 168, 159 S.E. 350 (1931)
12. Jordan Marsh Co. v. Cohen, 242 Mass. 245, 136 N.E. 350 (1922)
13. Hoard v. Gilbert, 205 Wis. 557, 238 N.W. 371 (1931)
14. McNaghten's Case, 10 Cl. & Fin. 200, 8 Eng. Rep. 718 (1843); Barnes; A Century of the McNaghten Rules. 8 *Camb. L. J.* 300 (1944)
15. The Law and the Mentally Ill. *Ment. Hygiene,* 53:4-40, Jan., 1969. The whole issue discusses various aspects of the topic. Penn, N.E., *et al.:* The Dilemma of Involuntary Commitment: Suggestions for a Measurable Alternative, pp. 4-9; Penn, N.E., *et al.:* Some Considerations for Future Mental Health Legislation, p. 10-13; Meyer, E. J.: Lawyer in a Mental Hospital, p. 14-16; Shah, S. A.: Crime and Mental Illness: Some Problems in Defining and Labeling Deviant Behavior

16. Durham v. United States, 94 App. D.C. 228, 214 F. 2d 862, motion denied 130 Fed. Supp. 445, 45 A.L.R. 2d 1430 (1954). There has been extensive comment on the case. See 53 *Mich. L. Rev.* 963 (1955); 18 *Modern L.R.* 391 (1955); 5 *Catholic U.L. Rev.* 63 (1955), and in the same issue, Cavanagh; "A Psychiatrist Looks at the Durham Decison," p. 25

17. Durrett v. McWhorter, 161 Ga. 179, 129 S.E. 870 (1925)

18. Dewey v. Algire, 37 Neb. 6, 55 N.W. 276 (1893); *In re* Herr's Estate, 251 Pa. 223, 96 Atl. 464 (1915); *In re* Halbert's Will, 15 Misc. 308, 37 N.Y.S. 757 (1895)

19. *In re* Wetmore, 6 Wash. 271, 33 Pac. 615 (1893)

20. Snyder v. Nixon, 188 Iowa 779, 176 N.W. 808 (1920)

21. Janneu v. Housekeeper, 70 Md. 162, 16 A.382 (1889)

22. Reid, Ronald L.: Birth Control Pills for Minors. *J. Med. Assn. Georgia,* 57:149-50, Mar., 1968

23. 1 Williston, Contracts, rev. ed. 1936, Sec. 238

24. Bishop v. Shurley, 237 Mich. 76, 211 N.W. 75 (1926)

25. Brockway v. Jewell, 52 Ohio St. 187, 39 N.E. 470 (1894)

General References

Creighton, Helen: Careful, That's A Contract! I. *RN, A Journal for Nurses,* 20 (11): 70-73, 82, Nov., 1957

— — —: Careful, That's A Contract! II. *RN., A Journal for Nurses,* 20 (12): 69-72, Dec., 1957

— — —: O.R. Nurses and the Law. *AORN Journal,* 4:65-72, 100-109, Mar.-Apr., 1966

Horty, John F.: Acceptance Rules Ensure Valid Contracts. *Mod. Hosp.,* 108:48-52, Mar., 1967

— — —: Contracts: What Constitutes a Valid Offer? *Mod. Hosp.,* 108:44-6, Apr., 1967

— — —: How Fraud Statutes Affect Oral Contracts. *Mod. Hosp.,* 108:58-62, May, 1967

— — —: Mutual Consent Is Basic Rule of Contracts. *Mod. Hosp.,* 108:58-63, Feb., 1967

— — —: What Are Rights of Contract Beneficiary? *Mod. Hosp.,* 108:52-4, June, 1967

Chapter Four

Breach and Termination of Contract

After an agreement has been made between two or more persons capable of contracting who create or intend to create a legal obligation, it is important for the nurse to consider how such a valid contract may be ended.

HOW TO TERMINATE A VALID CONTRACT

Obviously, one way of terminating a contract is for each person to duly *carry out all obligations* in accordance with the contract. Further, the contract may be ended by the release of one person by the other person. Sometimes a contract may be ended by the contracting person's agreeing to *substitute a new obligation or new person.* Of particular importance to nurses is the fact that although you can generally *assign or transfer your rights* to receive money under a contract without the consent of the other persons, you cannot transfer or assign duties of a personal nature unless this is acceptable to other persons to the contract. The contract may also provide for termination on the *expiration of a fixed period or the occurrence of a particular event.*

UNENFORCEABLE CONTRACTS

A contract may become unenforceable because suits on it are not brought within the time limit fixed in the *Statute of Limitations.* Contracts may also be ended because a supervening event makes performance *impossible.* In general, a person is excused from carrying out his obligation or duty in any contract when, through no fault of his own, such performance is *legally or physically impossible.* This is the situation in which a nurse is ill or dies, or her patient (on a private duty case) passes away. However, in a case in which a patient paid a physician in advance for treatments to be received, but became too ill to attend the physician's office for the treatments, the physician, having incurred no preparatory expense prior to the patient's disability, was required to return the money paid.[1] If the case had involved a nurse, instead of a physician, under similar circumstances, it is believed that the court would have reached the same result.

Again, if a nurse is prevented from carrying out her contractual obligations by some supervening event or *"act of God,"* such as a storm or a labor strike, she is excused in the majority of states. Inasmuch as the law is not uniform in all states on this question, the nurse will notice that written contracts often contain a sentence specifically providing for nonliability for performance when performance is impossible. At this point, the nurse is reminded that inconvenience and personal matters other than illness or death do not constitute a legal excuse for failure to carry out a contract. For example, consider the predicament of a nurse, Miss Jones, who lives in a suburb where public transportation facilities are limited and uses her own car for transportation to work. She accepts a position on a monthly basis at Hospital A in the downtown area of a large city. Subsequently, her car is destroyed, and she cannot afford to buy another one for three months. Now it takes Miss Jones 90 minutes instead of 20 minutes to get to work. By riding to work with a neighbor, Miss Jones can save an hour, but she arrives at the hospital 15 minutes late for duty. Nevertheless, Miss Jones decides that this is the only "sensible course of action," and she simply comes to work 15 minutes late. Such tardiness is a breach of contract.

Again, a married nurse, Mrs. Jones, whose two pre-school children are cared for by a maid "living out," accepts a position to work from 7:30 A.M. to 4 P.M. Monday through Friday at Hospital A. One Tuesday morning Mrs. Jones' maid calls and says, "I'm getting married and I'm taking off the rest of the week." Mrs. Jones stays home from her hospital position and cares for her children until her maid returns to work. Any nurse who foresees that circumstances will prevent her from carrying out a contract should point them out to the other person to the contract, and reserve the right to stop work or adjust her schedule if necessary. If she fails to do this, and does not perform her services, the hospital may regard the contract as ended. Furthermore, if the hospital sustains a money loss as a result thereof, it may consider the nurse as having broken the contract.

ILLEGAL CONTRACTS

Illegality excuses a nurse from carrying out a contract, as when the subject of the contract is declared illegal.

Contracts in Violation of the Law

For example, suppose a nurse, Miss Jones, makes a contract with Hospital A to serve as head nurse, and when on duty to start intravenous infusions on patients and to draw blood for various laboratory tests as ordered when no physician is available. In the event that the state in which Hospital A is located passes a law making it illegal for anyone except a duly licensed physician to do a venipuncture, Miss Jones' performance of her contract is excused.

Consent Obtained by Fraud

In the discussion of the requirement of a legally enforceable contract, it was pointed out that the real consent of the parties is necessary, and that no enforceable obligation is incurred if there is actually no expression of intention.[2] To constitute fraud, there must be a false representation of fact made with the intent that it be acted on by the other party, and such fact must be an inducing cause of the contract. For example, Nursing School C lists an opening for a qualified instructor in nursing fundamentals. A nurse, Miss Jones, makes application for the position and submits, as her own, certain transcripts of university undergraduate and graduate education and published educational articles, all the work of a person with the same name. In view of her apparent education and ability, Nursing School C employs Miss Jones for the position. The fraud in this so-called contract is apparent; a false representation of fact with the intent that it be acted on, and such fact is clearly an inducing element of the contract. In a case involving a physician in which the question of fraud arose, the court said that irrespective of the question of lack of benefit, a practitioner who by false representations as to the physical condition of his patient induces the patient to contract for his services will be denied the right to payment and will be compelled to refund any money paid to him for unnecessary treatment as a result of such fraud.[3]

Duress

Duress is another matter that will negate real consent of persons to a contract. At common law, duress means actual or threatened violence or imprisonment to the person or his wife, parent or child which is brought about by the other contracting party at the time that they make the contract. According to principles established in equity, the branch of law applying ethical or moral standards to disputes, contracts are considered voidable when brought about by forms of coercion and pressure which did not amount to duress at common law. The act complained of must be wrongful to cause duress. For example, in a suit on an agreement in which one contracting party, A, agreed to pay the husband, contracting party B, for medical treatment of his wife, who was injured by the negligence of the son of party A, in consideration of the husband's promise not to sue the son, the court stated that the husband's threats to start a law suit against the son did not amount to "duress." The court said that threat to exercise a legal right does not constitute "duress,"[4] even if the claims on which such suit was threatened were unfounded and the husband knew it.

Undue Influence

When a person is moved by undue influence to make a contract, it may be set aside. For example, an attractive young nurse with a "world of personality" is caring for an 86-year-old patient with a fractured hip when his recovery is interrupted by a stroke. As soon as the patient can talk a little and can use his hand to sign his name, the nurse calls in an attorney and has the patient make a will. In his will, the patient gives half of his property to the nurse. Ten days later, the patient dies. In such a case, the decedent's heirs are likely to question the validity of the will.

Material Misrepresentation

Aside from fraud, a material (significant) misrepresentation does away with real consent and may permit a person to avoid or cancel a contract. For example, if a private duty nurse, Miss Jones, has been engaged to care for a patient represented to her as a surgical case, a colostomy, and the patient is found to be a schizophrenic, Miss Jones may refuse to go on the case. She would not be liable for breach of contract, since there was no real consent, due to material misrepresentation. For misrepresentation to excuse performance, it must be of such importance that a reasonable person, had he known the situation, would not have made the contract, indicating that the person who desires to negate the contract was in fact misled.

Mistake

Mistake is another matter preventing real consent in the formation of a contract. In general, the question of "mistake" is a difficult one. Obviously, ignorance of a fact is not enough to permit canceling the contract. For example, Mr. Smith contracts with Miss Jones for a week's nursing service to be given to his best friend, Mr. Doe. He is bound by the contract even though he did not read it before signing. There may be mistake as to the identity of a contracting person and mistake concerning the subject matter.

DISCRIMINATION

The recent trend has been to outlaw discrimination on the basis of race, creed, color or national origin. A state statute requiring segregation of passengers on railroads was held to be valid and nondiscriminatory if equal facilities were at the disposal of each racial group in 1896.[5] Fifty years later, the requirement of segregated seating for passengers on interstate buses was held to be unconstitutional. By 1950, racial segregation was enjoined in a state university[6] and segregated city-owned recreational facilities, even though equal, were prohibited.[7] More recently, school desegregation rulings, public accommodation statutes, employment regulations, open housing laws and so forth are aimed at eliminating all discrimination insofar as the law can achieve it.

When a unit of government operates a hospital, it must be open to all citizens on the same basis. For many years, a charitable hospital has been open:

> . . . at the call of the afflicted . . . looking at nothing and caring
> for nothing beyond the fact of their affliction.[8]

Other states have for years required of a hospital, to be tax-exempt, that it accept patients without discrimination as to race, creed or color.[9] When the guardian of a severely retarded Negro child sued a state mental institution to enjoin it from denying him admission on racial grounds, the action against the hospital was dismissed when it proved it did routinely admit Negro patients but could not accept him because of 100 per cent occupancy of all accommodations it had.[10]

When Negro physicians and their patients brought action against a hospital for denying admission to staff membership and treatment facilities on a racially discriminatory and segregated basis, the court held that the hospital was performing the state's function and was a chosen instrument of the state, and that accordingly it was bound by the fourteenth amendment to refrain from the alleged discrimination.[11] The growing use of Federal funds in hospital administration brings with it the sanctions of the Civil Rights Act of 1964.[12]

BREACH OF CONTRACT

Consideration has been given to means whereby a contract may be terminated and situations which legally excuse the performance of a contract for personal services. Attention is directed to what is meant by breach of contract. If one person to a personal service contract does not perform his obligations as required under it, he commits a breach of contract unless his performance has been excused on one of the grounds noted.

Remedies

Although there are three remedies for breach of contract,[13] usually the nurse is concerned with only one, damages.

Damages. "Damages" is a term referring to a sum of money awarded to one person because another has disregarded his rights as established by law.[14] Damages are given if it is shown that the breach of contract caused money loss to the person who complains.[15] In addition to damages, when there is a material breach of contract, the injured person may choose to reject the contract, provided that the breach "goes to the root of the contract." Specific performance is not ordered in such personal service contracts. Nor is it likely that a court would issue an order prohibiting the doing of an act causing a breach of contract for nursing service.

Definition of Right and of Remedy at Law

What do the terms "right" and "remedy at law" mean? Perhaps a nurse is told that she has certain rights under the law. The term "right" is defined to mean that which a person is entitled to have or do, or to receive from another, whose duty is imposed within the limits prescribed by law.[16] As concerns contracts, there exists the right to performance or to sue for a broken contract. Therefore a nurse needs to know what rights arise in various situations.

A remedy is the means by which a right is enforced, or the violation of a right is prevented.* As pointed out earlier, there are several remedies for breach of contract. The party injured by a breach of contract has a right to damages for the loss suffered. Thus, when a breach of contract happens, if the injured party has done a portion but not all of what he was obliged to do by the contract, he can claim the value of what he has done. In certain circumstances, an injured party may get a decree of specific performance of the contract or an injunction to prevent its breach. This remedy is inapplicable to contracts for nursing service.

---

*Judge Cothran said: "A remediable right is a legal conclusion from certain stated facts; a remedy is the appropriate legal form of relief by which that remediable right may be enforced."[17]

Examples of Breach of Contract

Failure to fulfill terms of contract. Suppose that a nurse was engaged by a hospital, and that among other benefits she was promised a private room and laundry service, neither of which she received. This would be a failure on the part of the hospital to carry out its part of the agreement, and hence it may be said to have breached the contract by not having fully lived up to its obligations.

Again, suppose that a nurse was employed by a Visiting Nurse Association at a salary of $625.00 a month, with a month's paid vacation after one year's employment, and a mileage allowance of seven cents per mile for use of her car when used in line of duty. The nurse worked for the Visiting Nurse Association for six months, during which time she was required to use her car in answering calls. The association paid her salary, but did not reimburse her for the use of her car on its business. The nurse may enforce her right to damages for breach of contract.

Misrepresentation. If a private duty nurse has been engaged to care for a patient and there has been a misrepresentation, knowingly or unknowingly, as to the nature of the case, she may refuse to enter duty, and she will not be liable for breach of contract, as in the example in which the patient was stated to be a surgical case when in fact he was also a patient with a severe mental disorder. The nurse may sue for damages if she sustains a money loss because of her inability to obtain another case immediately. On the other hand, if the nurse has rendered some service on the contract before she discovers the misrepresentation, she may terminate the contract at once and recover damages for services given. If she continues on the case, the law looks upon her continuation as an agreement on her part to waive the effect of misrepresentation. However, the nurse is somewhat "on the spot." When a nurse has started to give care to a patient before finding out the real situation, she must give the patient time to get another nurse, and she must be careful not to neglect the patient so as to place him in a less favorable condition.

Negligence. In the performance of her services, a nurse is required to use "due care." She would be responsible if a patient breaks his leg as a result of falling out of bed while delirious because the nurse left him unattended for five minutes while she had a cigarette and a Coke. Damages would be his earnings for loss of time at work had he returned to work sooner plus hospital and medical bills. This is nothing more than a modern version of the old statement that:

> It is the duty of every artificer to exercise his art right and truly as he ought.[18]

As the court has stated in a modern case:

> It is a sound rule of law that one who, by reason of his professional relation is placed in a position where it becomes his

duty to exercise ordinary care to protect others from injury or danger is liable in damages to those who are injured by reason of his failure to exercise such care.[19]

In this connection, it is pointed out that when a nurse is caring for a patient and his safety requires one in attendance, she is bound to use "due care" and to remain until provision is made for his safety. This is true even if she has finished her hours of duty as expressed in her employment contract.

TYPES OF ACTIONS BROUGHT AGAINST NURSES

Injuries Due to Negligence or Wrongful Act

The nurse should give some thought to the type of action which may be brought against her by one seeking compensation for injuries due to a negligent or wrongful act on her part.[20] The persons involved in a lawsuit are the plaintiff,[21] the one who starts an action to obtain a remedy for an injury to his rights, and the defendant, who is required to make answer and defend the action or lose by default. The plaintiff's complaint (declaration) has to show a right based upon the relationship between plaintiff and defendant, a corresponding duty to the plaintiff imposed upon the defendant by the relationship, a violation of the right and duty, the resulting injury to the plaintiff.[22]

The relation between nurse and patient may arise out of contract, as in the case of a private duty nurse. Therefore, a patient who has suffered injury through the negligence of such a nurse may sue on the basis of the contract, alleging a breach of the contract by which the nurse undertook to care for him with due (ordinary) care and skill, as a result of which he has sustained a monetary (pecuniary) loss. However, it is well for the nurse to realize that, if the patient wishes, when the provisions of the contract are broken, he may bring action arising directly out of the breach of duty created by the contract. Or, again, the plaintiff may rely on negligence, simply stating that the defendant has breached the legal duty to use care, resulting in injury to the plaintiff, for which he asks damages.

DEFINITION OF TORT

The nurse is reminded that choosing the type of action is a practical matter of some consequence. The type of action brought often determines the length of time allowed before it must be commenced by filing a complaint in court. A tort is a legal wrong committed upon the person or property independent of contract. It may be either a direct invasion of some legal right of the person, the infraction of some public duty by which special damage accrues to the person, or the violation of some private obligation by which like damage accrues to the person.[23] For example, if State A has a statute saying that actions for breach of contract may be brought within six years and actions for "tort resulting in personal injury" must be started within two years, the length of time between the injury and the starting of the action is important. If a plaintiff sues in a tort action three years after receiving injuries entitling him to damages, the statute of limitations would be a good defense and bar compensation. On the other hand, such a plaintiff might have a good action on the contract.[24] It is also important to determine in such a situation whether the court considers the action properly based on a breach of contract rather than a violation of a duty commanded by law. If a nurse should become involved in a case, she should find out the rule of her jurisdiction, since there is some difference of opinion among the courts. Once an issue is determined on its merits by a court having proper jurisdiction, its judgment is a bar to any further litigation upon the same matter by the same persons. This rule of law is known as *res adjudicata.*

As previously pointed out, a contract for nursing services is a contract which is personal in nature. The personal services must be given by the nurse making the contract and not by a substitute nurse. For example, Mr. Smith engages a nurse, Miss Jones, to care for him after a heart attack. After working seven days a week for four weeks, Miss Jones feels the need of "time off" duty and sends Miss Doe, an equally experienced and skillful nurse, to care for Mr. Smith in her place. When the contract contains no provision for a substitute nurse, a breach of contract occurs if a substitute is provided without the consent of the patient. Preventing a person from carrying out a personal service contract, such as one for nursing services, would also constitute a breach of such contract.

UNENFORCEABLE CONTRACTS EXPLAINED

Although primarily concerned with legal contracts, the nurse must be aware that attempts may be made to form unenforceable contracts. Let it be clear that no remedies are provided by law for breach of illegal contracts.

Examples

For example, suppose that a nurse, Miss Jones, promises in exchange for $30.00 to obtain six ampules of Demerol from a hospital for a man, Mr. Doe, who is a known drug addict. She delivers the Demerol to Mr. Doe, but he refuses to pay her. The law will not compel Mr. Doe to pay her. This contract violates the narcotic laws.

Another example would be that of a contract between Miss Jones, a nurse, and Dr. Doe to assist him in performing an illegal abortion on a patient. The law will not permit Miss Jones in such a case to collect her wages when Dr. Doe refuses to pay for her services. The contract is illegal and void. Contracts to obstruct justice, in fraud of creditors, and in excessive restraint of trade are also void, and no remedy may be had for breach of such contracts.

Again, a nurse must be careful not to diagnose diseases or ailments or to prescribe treatments for their relief for compensation; such matters commonly come within the practice of medicine or surgery. A nurse has no license to do these acts, and therefore she cannot make a valid contract to do them for compensation.[25] The same interpretation is placed upon the act of a nurse misrepresenting herself as a licensed nurse in a jurisdiction requiring a license. As the court has said in a number of cases, under statutes regulating the right to practice medicine, surgery, dentistry and similar professions, when there has been a failure to comply with the statutory requisites for admission, no recovery can be had for services rendered in a professional capacity.[26] It has been decided that money paid to an unlicensed practitioner may be recovered, at least as long as the agreement as to the services remains uncompleted.[27] However, a law prohibiting practice as a nurse, or engaging in the care of the sick as an attendant, without a license, does not prevent a recovery for the rendering of services in the nature of nursing as incidental to general employment as a caretaker.[28]

STATUTES OF LIMITATIONS ON DAMAGES

Before leaving unenforceable contracts, another feature must be discussed. If claims regarding breach of contract are presented after a long delay, the lapse of time may be pleaded as a defense. At (1623) common law, there was no specified time limit as to when a person having a cause of action was required to start suit. However, statutes of limitation differing somewhat in their terms have been passed in all states. If there are no express statutory provisions for malpractice actions, actions for damages from injury due to malpractice are governed by the limitations on actions for damages arising out of personal injuries. The time limitation varies in the different states, and ranges from two to six years. In the case of a contract it may depend, among other things, on whether it was a simple contract or a formal one in writing. The time when the statute begins to run is also important: whether from the date of the act causing injury or from the date of the discovery of the cause of injury.

Several recent court decisions show the courts' tendency to reckon the statute of limitations from the time of discovery rather than from the date the alleged malpractice was committed. In *Billings v. Sisters of Mercy,*[29] the patient, after undergoing an exploratory operation, sued to recover for damages arising from the discovery of a gauze sponge left in his body in an operation 15 years earlier; the court held that the statute of limitations did not bar the action. In *Rahn v. United States,*[30] a patient with a broken wrist was treated at an Air Force base hospital. When she complained that she was not able to use her hand, the physicians told her that her condition was progressing satisfactorily. Later, when the patient brought a suit against the United States Government for damages due to loss of the use of her hand, the Georgia two-year statute of limitations was held not to bar the action due to concealment of important facts during that period. Until the necessary facts were discovered, the statute did not start to run. In *Phelps v. Donaldson,*[31] a patient expressed dissatisfaction with an orthodontist's work. In that case, the one-year statute of limitations barred his suit when it was brought after that period.

In *Gross v. Wise,*[32] a patient sued a physician for malpractice for treatment that extended over a three-year-period. The court held the reckoning of the statute of limitations as starting from the time of the end of the treatment.

Since in some cities and states it may take four to six years before a personal injury suit comes to trial, the statute of limitations could expire and preclude recovery of medical bills even if the patient eventually wins his suit. This is a serious problem, for the patient's capability of paying for medical care he received after being injured often is based upon a court's award of damages. A way to protect the hospital's and physician's interests was found by a New York physician who obtained an assignment of an appropriate portion of anticipated damages from his patient as security for payment for treating him after an accident. The physician then notified the defendant's insurer. The physician ultimately secured his money, since his assignment had not ripened into a legal claim until the settlement of the lawsuit.[33]

During the time that a patient is insane, the statute of limitations does not operate. In the case of a patient who suffered postoperative brain damage and who sued a physician after his mental recovery, the court said that the person who is insane at the time of the claimed malpractice has the full statutory period after the disability is removed to bring a suit.

Under most statutes of limitation, if a person leaves the jurisdiction or fraudulently hides himself so that he cannot be served a summons, the time limit for an action may be extended. If the person responsible for negligence or breach of contract dies, proceedings should be started against the personal representative authorized to act for the estate of the deceased within the period allowed by statute.

The statute of limitations is directed at barring the remedy and not the commencement of actions to recover. Therefore, most statutes permit recovery on contract claims after the expiration of the time limit when a person makes a payment or signs a paper acknowledging his debt. For a summary of the statute of limitations in each state, see reference 34 of this chapter.

If the relation between nurse and patient arises out of contract, it follows that the nurse's right to salary or wages is governed by the same contract. The performance of duty owed by the nurse, to give nursing services to the patient, must be shown to entitle her to receive payment for such services. Failure to pay a nurse for services in accordance with the contract is a breach of contract for which a nurse may sue.

REFERENCES

1. Bucklin v. Morton, 105 Misc. 46, 172 N.Y.S. 344 (1918)
2. Anson, William R.: *Principles of the English Law of Contract and of Agency in Its Relation to Contract*, 20th ed., 1952, p. 144
3. Barker v. Weeks, 182 Wash. 384, 47 P. 2d 1 (1935)
4. Plunkett v. O'Connor, 162 Misc. 839, 295 N.Y.S. 492 (1937)
5. Plessy v. Ferguson, 163 U.S. 537, 16 S. Ct. 1138, 41 L. Ed. 256 (1896)
6. Morgan v. Virginia, 328 U.S. 373, 66 S. Ct. 1050, 90 L. Ed. 1317 (1946)
7. McLaurin v. Oklahoma State Regents, 339 U.S. 637, 70 S. Ct. 851, 94 L. Ed. 1149 (1950)
8. Schloendorff v. The Society of the New York Hospital, 211 N.Y. 625, 105 N.E. 92 (1914)
9. San Antonio v. Santa Rosa Infirmary, 259 S.W. 926 (Tex., 1924)
10. Johnson v. Crawfis, 128 F. Supp. 230 (Ark., 1955)
11. Eaton *et al.* v. Grubbs and Board of Managers of James Walker Memorial Hospital, 329 F. 2d 710 (N.C., 1964)
12. Cypress *et al.* v. Newport News General and Non-Sectarian Hospital Assn., 251 F. Supp. 667 (1966)
13. Williston: *Contracts,* rev. ed. 1936, p. 683-688
14. Prosser: *Torts.* Hornbook, 1955, § 2; Morris: Punitive Damage in Tort Cases. 44 Harv. L. Rev. 1173 (1931); Simpson: *Handbook of the Law of Contracts.* Hornbook, 1955, §§ 148-157; Rubin: May a Person Be Convicted of a Felony and Yet Escape Civil Liability Therefore?" 10 Marq. L. Rev. 113 (1926)
15. McQuaid v. Michou, 85 N.H. 299, 157 Atl. 881 (1932); Burns v. American Nat. Ins. Co., 280 S.W. 762 (Tex. Civ. App., 1936)
16. Atchison & N.R. Co. v. Baty, 6 Neb. 37, 29 Am. Rep. 356 (1877). See also Coke: *2 Institutes of the Laws of England;* or a Commentary upon Littleton, 1812, *345 (a)
17. Ebner v. Haverty Furniture Co., 138 S.C. 74, 136 S.E. 19 (1926)
18. Fitzherbert: *Natura Brevium,* 94 D. 208 D (1534)
19. Davis v. Rodman, 147 Ark. 385, 227 S.W. 612 (1921)
20. Singely v. Bigelow, 108 Cal. App. 436, 291 Pac. 899 (1930)
21. Pomeroy: *Code Remedies,* 5th ed. 1929, §§ 62-81
22. *Ibid.,* § 2
23. Prosser, op. cit. supra, § 1; Stone; Touchstones of Tort Liability, 2 *Stan. L. Rev.* 259 (1950); Radin: A Speculative Inquiry into the Nature of Torts. 21 *Texas L. Rev.* 697 (1943)
24. Boane v. Austin, 156 Tenn. 353, 2 S.W. 2d 100 (1928)
25. People *ex rel.* Burke v. Steinberg, 73 N.Y.S. 2d 475 (N.Y.C. Mag. Ct. 1947)
26. Whitehead v. Coker, 16 Ala. App. 165, 76 So. 484 (1917); Rubin v. Douglas, 59 A

2nd 690 (D.C. Munic. Ct. 1948); Hoxsey v. Baker, 216 Iowa 85, 246 N.W. 653 (1933); Katsafaros v. Agathakos, 52 Ohio App. 290, 3 N.E. 2d 810 (1935)

27. Deaton v. Lawson, 40 Wash. 486, 82 P. 879, 2 L.R.A. (N.S.) 392 (1935)
28. Marker v. Cleveland, 212 Mo. App. 467, 252 S.W. 95 (1923); see Physicians and Surgeons, 48 C.J. 1159, § 168, n. 59, Failure to register or record license; see also "Witnesses," 70 C.J.S. 1027, § 1225, Asking or examining witnesses as to inconsistent or contradictory statements.
29. Billings v. Sisters of Mercy of Idaho, 86 Ida. 485, 389 P. 2d 224 (1964)
30. Rahn v. United States, 42 A. 2d 200, 80 A. 2d 368, 222 F. Suff. 775 (1963)
31. Phelps v. Donaldson, 243 La. 1118, 150 So. 2d 35 (S.Ct. of La., 1963)
32. Gross v. Wise, 18A Đ 1097, 227, N.Y.S. 2d 523 239 N.Y.S. 2d 954 (1963)
33. Bernstein v. Allstate Insurance Co., 228 N.Y.S. 2d 646 (Civ. Ct. N.Y.C., 1968)
34. Creighton, Helen: O.R. Nurses and the Law. *AORN Journal,* 4:65-72, 100-109, Mar.-Apr., 1966

Chapter Five

The Legal Status of the Nurse

TYPES OF RELATIONSHIPS WHEN SERVICES ARE PERFORMED

The relationship between parties whereby one person, such as a nurse, performs services for another person in various situations may fix the limitations of liability in a legal action to recover damages caused by wrongful or negligent acts. The existence of a certain relationship may also determine whether a certain person is entitled to rights and benefits given to "employees" by various federal and state laws. It follows that the meanings of the terms "employer" and "employee" are important. In some employment situations a nurse may be an employee, while in others she may be an independent contractor, and it is important for her to know the difference. In general, when one person performs services for another, the parties in various relationships may be classified under the headings employer and employee, and employer and independent contractor.

EMPLOYER AND EMPLOYEE

Again, the nurse is reminded that each person is personally liable for negligent acts.[1] In addition, an employee may make the employer liable as well. In the latter case a person injured by an

55

employee's negligent act may be able to bring an action against both employer and employee and thereby increase his chance of collecting. The person injured by an employee's negligent act may not collect twice for the same injury, but he may bring actions against separate defendants. Because it is not always possible to make a clear-cut test of a relationship, the nurse needs to know the factors involved.

Definition of Terms

Generally speaking, the employer is the person who has the "right to control" and direct another in the performance of the work, including the details and means by which the work is to be done. It is not necessary that the employer actually direct or control the way in which the services are done; it is enough that he, as employer, is legally entitled to do so.[2]

In a doubtful case, the relationship has to be determined in the light of the facts. In a negligence case brought against a surgeon operating on a patient, *the surgeon was held not liable* when injury resulted to the patient because a scrub nurse at the hospital had used a different machine from the one the surgeon ordered. The court expressed the opinion that the scrub nurse, in setting up the operating room, was not an employee of the surgeon, since the hospital could direct how such work should be done.[3] A different relationship exists when a nurse is supplied by the hospital to assist the surgeon in an operation.[4] Then it is the duty of the surgeon, in using the nurse furnished by the hospital, to see that every act necessary for the operation and under his supervision is properly done. In such a case, the nurse is working under the surgeon's orders; he controls her acts, and thereby the surgeon becomes the employer.

A person becomes an employee, generally speaking, when he performs services for another who has the "right to control" what is done and how it is to be done. An employee is one who works for wages or salary in the service of an employer. The power to discharge is that of the employer,[5] although in some instances this is modified by law. As the Social Security Act points out, other factors characteristic of an employer are the furnishing of tools and a place to work to the person who performs the services. It is important to realize that the controlling factor is the relationship which actually exists, and not the terms by which the persons are described.

Student Nurses as Employees

The student nurse is usually an employee, since she is subject to the control of clinical instructors, head nurses, and physicians. The element of control by head nurses, supervisors and physicians may also apply to other classifications of nurses. As an employee, the student nurse in carrying out her duties must act as a reasonably prudent person under the circumstances, and the amount of experience and education, her record and grades are some of the matters considered. Responsibility increases as a nurse progresses in professional knowledge and experience. It is well to remember that anyone who undertakes to act as a nurse becomes subject to duties, so that failure to perform them may constitute negligence.[6] In the student nurse's educational program, she is assigned to practical ward duty for experience, and courts have held that when so assigned she is performing services for the hospital, and therefore the hospital is her employer. For example, in an emergency during an influenza epidemic, two student nurses received the head nurse's permission to give nursing care during off-duty hours. The parent of a child patient who was burned by a lighted alcohol inhalator brought suit; the court, in holding that the hospital and the student nurses were liable for actual damage resulting from their negligence, said that the student nurses were acting within the scope of their employment in caring for the child.[7]

Social Security Act of 1950

The Social Security Act of 1950 defined employees for purposes of the Act, and specifically excepted certain nurses by the following from its provisions:

> ... services performed as a student nurse in the employ of a hospital or nurses' training school by an individual who is enrolled and is regularly attending classes in a nurses' training school chartered or approved pursuant to state law.[8]

The 1950 amendment to the Social Security Act permits voluntary participation by employees of nonprofit hospitals and employees of state and municipal hospitals and convalescent homes.[9] Participation in the Social Security program depends upon the decision of the Hospital Board and requests therefor by two-thirds of the employees at the time of election. Since no class of nurses has been explicitly excluded, private duty nurses are considered eligible to take part in the voluntary program.

Workmen's Compensation Laws

Workmen's Compensation Laws, with some exceptions, provide for a fixed schedule of benefits and medical benefits to employees or their dependents in case of industrial accidents or disease.[10] "Workmen" has the same meaning as employees. Hence, the nurse is interested in determining whether she qualifies under such legislation. First, the nurse has to know whether she is an employee, and next, whether her employer comes within the coverage of the compensation law. The Workmen's Compensation Laws do away with the requirement of proof that the employer was negligent or that the employee was free from contributory negligence.

In *Denver v. Pollard*,[11] a public health nurse employed by the City and County of Denver worked in close proximity to patients infected with beta streptococcus. When she became infected, suffered from rheumatic fever and as a result was forced to leave her work, she brought suit before the Industrial Commission to obtain weekly compensation. It was granted.

Likewise, the defenses of assumption of risk and negligence of a fellow employee are eliminated. Also, Workmen's Compensations Acts prevent court actions for injuries and provide instead a simple administrative procedure for securing awards of compensation. In many states, government employees (for example, nurses) are not eligible under Workmen's Compensation Laws, but are covered under the Federal Employees Compensation Act.[12] Many Workmen's Compensation Laws exclude casual employees; hence private duty nurses employed on different cases for short periods are generally not eligible.

The meaning of the assumption of risk doctrine is illustrated by the case of a practical nurse engaged by the wife of a patient in Doctors Hospital and Clinic. After the patient had gone to the bathroom alone, he was heard calling for assistance in a weak voice. The nurse responded and was assisting him back to bed when her leg twisted and the patient fell on her, and she suffered a depressed fracture of the leg. The practical nurse sued the hospital for damages, claiming it had been negligent. The court of appeals ruled in favor of the hospital and applied the doctrine of assumption of the risk in this case.[13]

In some states, the Workmen's Compensation Law is compulsory, and every employer belonging to designated groups must accept it. In other states, the Workmen's Compensation Law is elective, and both employer and employee can accept or reject its coverage. When the law is elective, the employer may provide employees with the benefits under the law by posting bond with the state and becoming a self-insurer or by getting an insurance policy therefor. When a hospital does not come within the Workmen's Compensation Law, an injured employee, such as a nurse, is in the same position as any other person who is not covered. The nurse should make it her business to know her status in regard to the Workmen's Compensation Laws in her state.

EXPLANATION OF "MASTER-SERVANT RULE"

The "master-servant rule" (*respondeat superior*) makes a master responsible for the wrongful acts of his servant, in certain cases, and the same rule applies to the relationship of a principal and agent. For example, whenever a person is injured by an employee as a result of negligence in the course of the employee's work, the employer is responsible to the injured person. In this situation, the injured person may sue both the employee and employer, and hence has a better chance of being compensated for his injury. However, a double recovery is not allowed.

It is pointed out that the relationship of employer and employee is not negated by the fact that the employee is doing work of a technical or highly skilled nature which the employer could not do himself.

> The aviation company which employs an aviator to fly an aeroplane on a difficult course is liable for his negligence. . . . Similarly, a steamship company is liable for the negligence of the certified shipmasters who are navigating its ships. In such cases, the employers are liable, even though they cannot tell their servants how to perform the tasks they have employed them to do, and would, in fact, make themselves criminally liable if they attempted to do so.[14]

The significance of this theory is apparent in connection with claims against hospitals.

EMPLOYER AND INDEPENDENT CONTRACTOR

The law defines an independent contractor as a person contracting with another to do something for him, but not controlled by the other, nor subject to the other's "right to control" with respect to his physical conduct in the performance of the undertaking (work or service).[15] Applying this definition to the nurse, it becomes apparent that if a nurse is subject to control of another merely as to the result of the work, and not as to the means by which the result is reached, she may be an independent contractor.

Private Duty Nurses as Independent Contractors

Most of the nurses who are in this class are professional nurses acting as private duty nurses. If the nurse is regarded as an independent contractor, she is answerable for any wrong she may commit, and the hospital in which she is working is not liable. For example, in an action by a patient to recover for burns occurring after an operation, it was shown that these burns were caused by electric pads put on the patient by a special duty nurse, and the hospital was held not liable. Here, the acts causing the injury occurred as a part of the professional treatment by one not subject to control or direction by the administrative officers of the hospital.[16]

Again, it is said that when the patient engages a nurse as a special duty nurse, she is an independent contractor and is legally responsible for fulfilling her duties.[17] In a New York case, this question arose in a law suit over injury to the patient, and the nurse was held liable as an independent contractor,[18] although the hospital paid the nurse and collected from the patient. It seems to be a general rule that a hospital is not responsible by contract or in tort for acts of surgeons, physicians or special nurses who take care of patients in the hospital.[19]

There is also some authority that in an ordinary case in which the nurse performs her usual duties with the skill resulting from her training in the profession, she is not considered an employee in the usual sense, but one who renders personal service to an employer in pursuit of an independent calling.[20]

Agent as Employee or Independent Contractor

An agent may be an employee or an independent contractor, depending upon the type of relationship entered into with his principal. Thus, an agent would be an independent contractor if he is engaged in an independent trade, business or occupation and agrees to perform his work or services with no control by the principal over the way in which the details are carried out. However, at any one time a person cannot be both an employee and an independent contractor.

Liability of the Supervising Nurse for Negligence of Others

As the profession of nursing continues to grow, the professional registered nurse is having to assume more and more responsibility for supervising the work of others: graduate nurses, student nurses, practical nurses, and others who help the patient. In this connection, it is pointed out that a supervising nurse may be liable for the negligence* of others, that is, of persons to whom she has assigned certain duties. For example, when a nurse supervisor failed to call a physician for three days when a general duty nurse reported that a patient recovering from an operation showed signs of pathology, the supervising nurse was held liable.[22] The law requires that each person act with ordinary (due) care towards other persons. That means the care which would be used by an average, careful nurse supervisor. To illustrate further, judgment for damages was entered against a

---

*In *Blyth v. Birmingham Waterworks Co.*[21] Judge Alderson stated: "Negligence is the omission to do something which a reasonable man, guided upon those considerations which ordinarily regulate the conduct of human affairs, would do or do something which a prudent and reasonable man would not do."

supervising nurse in charge of unused sponges in surgery when it appeared that death of the patient was due to an infection arising from a sponge left in the abdomen. The evidence showed that the person to whom the count was left was not competent without immediate supervision, which was lacking.[23]

In the event that a registered nurse assigns a student or practical nurse to duties beyond her ability to carry out, and negligence occurs, the registered nurse is responsible. This rule is based on the fact that she should not assign the duties which she knows or should know the person selected is incompetent to perform because of inexperience or insufficient education. In other words, she should not assign duties that such a person could perform only under adequate supervision and then fail to provide the supervision, in accordance with the standard of care used by an average, careful supervisor in similar circumstances.

Rights of the Private Duty Nurse in a Hospital

The private duty nurse or other nurse who is serving as an independent contractor in a hospital has certain rights and may expect certain conditions from the hospital. In order that such a nurse may render proper service to her patient, she can expect the hospital to supply suitable and necessary equipment. Moreover, the nurse can rightfully expect the hospital to keep its premises and equipment in a reasonably safe condition. She may also expect that the hospital will require of its employees reasonable care in their work.[24] If the nurse suffers injury because of failure of the hospital to provide suitable conditions, recovery on her claim may be prevented if the hospital is a charitable institution. This problem will be discussed in the paragraphs which follow.

"Let the Master Answer" Explained

"Let the master answer" (*respondeat superior*) is a principle of law making an employer liable for damages caused by a wrongful act of his servant within the scope of his employment. For example, in a Georgia hospital, a newborn baby who needed a blood change-over operation was strapped in an incubator by nurses for surgery. Due to error, one of the baby's feet rested against a bare light bulb used to heat the incubator, and as a result of the burns she lost the major portion of her foot. The defendant hospital was held liable for the negligence of its nurse employees.[25]

A physician, too, has been held liable in a $25,000 judgment when an office nurse's report slowed therapy and the patient died.[26] The toddler had been seen by the physician that morning, at which time his condition was diagnosed and he was treated with antibiotics.

Some two hours later the mother returned with the boy and told the nurse she thought he had convulsions and was dying. The physician was at lunch, and the nurse called him to report what the mother said, but added that she (the nurse) thought his condition was about the same as earlier in the morning. Leaving the receptionist in charge, the nurse also went to lunch. Some minutes later the little boy lying on the examining table vomited and his respirations became scarcely visible. Although the receptionist called the physician, he arrived after the boy had died. At trial, there was a preponderance of evidence that the probable cause of death was the negligence of the nurse.

It is pointed out that in view of this doctrine, a nurse shortage can be risky to the hospital. At law, the standard of care requires sufficient nursing service personnel to meet the apparent physical needs of the patient. When nurses from other countries are utilized, when student nurses are used as registered professional nurses, and when the number of nursing aides and practical nurses is much greater than the number of registered professional nurses (as happens many times on evenings and nights), the hospital should realize that the doctrine of *respondeat superior* (the employer answers for the employee) applies to all hospitals and all hospital employees.[27] The employer is not responsible when he employs an independent contractor to act for him unless there are special circumstances, as when the employer fails to use proper care in selecting a competent contractor. The master will be liable also for acts of independent contractors when work done is "extra hazardous," e.g., the use of scaffolding to paint a building.

Liability of Hospitals

It is often difficult to decide whether a person employed by another is his servant or an independent contractor, and this question often arises in connection with the wrongful acts of nurses in hospitals. Generally speaking, the most important criterion in deciding this question is the "right to control" or supervise the details of performing the services.

Recovery for negligence is further complicated in the United States since hospitals are divided into three classes: public (government) hospitals, private nonprofit charitable hospitals and private hospitals run for profit (proprietary hospitals). The liability of a hospital as an employer varies with its classification. Since a nurse frequently practices her profession in a hospital, it is important for her to know the difference between a voluntary nonprofit charitable institution and the private profit-making hospital. The former type of hospital is far more numerous than the latter.

Immunity of charitable hospitals. A hospital operated as a "charitable" institution does not, of course, treat and care for patients free of charge. Such charitable hospitals may incidentally have free or nonpaying patients, but for the most part they charge standard fees for services rendered. Important factors in deciding the classification include the purpose of the hospital, the type of organization, and its character as set forth in the charter or articles of incorporation. In a charitable hospital, any funds over and above expenses usually go to the maintenance fund, for use on expansion of facilities or for research in health problems, so as to further the purposes of the institution.

The immunity of charitable institutions in cases of negligence of employees has been based on different theories: that public policy supports an immunity; that the assets of the institution, being impressed with a trust for a charitable purpose, may not be used otherwise; and that patients who voluntarily enter assume the risk and waive claims for injuries.[28] For example, in a state where a hospital as a charitable institution has immunity, a patient was unable to collect damage from a hospital for injuries resulting from a burn caused by a nurse's negligence in placing a hot water bottle.[29] But a charitable hospital was held liable to a paying patient when a student nurse who had been in training only seven months administered morphine, instead of a given dose of codeine, to a 6-year-old boy who had been apparently recovering from an operation, but who died as a result of the morphine.[30] In another type of case, a charitable hospital protected by liability insurance has been held liable for negligence in care and medical treatment.[31]

There is a conflict in the decisions of the various states as to whether or not the beneficiaries of the charity may recover for injuries due to negligence when it is not shown that there was negligence in selecting the employee.[32] For example, when a student nurse through negligence caused a severe burn on a patient, one court held that the only obligation a charitable institution owes either pay patients or charity patients is to select with reasonable care the persons who act as nurses.[33] Thus, the charitable hospital was liable on the basis of not using due and reasonable care in the selection of the employee when a patient brought an action for damages due to burns caused by a student's negligently administering a clysis of scalding hot water to a patient while he was under the influence of ether after an appendectomy.[34]

The nurse should note, however, that the trend of recent decisions is toward discarding the immunity rule and toward holding charitable institutions liable for the negligent acts of employees. This view was adopted when a private duty nurse suffered permanent injuries from a swinging door because of the negligence of a student nurse, the charitable hospital being held liable under the usual "master-servant rule."* In another case, in which a patient sued to recover for injuries received when he was thrown from a stretcher that was being moved by a nurse's aide who lost control over it, a charitable hospital was liable.[35] California, Minnesota and Arizona in decided cases have made the charitable hospital, as the employer, liable for the nurse's negligence.

The trend to limit the charitable immunity of voluntary nonprofit hospitals continues. The West Virginia Court has followed similar action taken recently by the Supreme Court of Pennsylvania, which held that a paying patient may sue a charitable institution for negligence. A partially paralyzed patient with impaired vision, who was being prepared by an orderly for a tub bath, fell against a steam radiator. While the orderly went for assistance, the patient remained on the hot radiator and sustained third degree burns. The patient claimed that the hospital was negligent in employing and retaining incompetent help and that, as a result, he was injured. The hospital claimed immunity from damage suits, but the court rejected the immunity claim.[36]

In another case, the charitable hospital was held liable in damages because it had no pharmacist. A child who had swallowed some pills was taken to the emergency room of the hospital, where the doctor ordered a 2-teaspoon dose of ipecac. The dose was administered from a bottle marked syrup of ipecac but the child soon died. Later, another child, to whom the same ipecac was given, also died. The medicine was fluid extract of ipecac instead of syrup of ipecac. The hospital did not employ a registered pharmacist in its pharmacy. The court held that the charitable immunity doctrine did not protect the appellee (hospital) from liability for damages for injuries caused by administrative negligence as to nondelegable duties.[37]

CIVIL RIGHTS ACT

The Civil Rights Act of 1964 forbids discrimination against any person on the grounds of race, color or national origin in relation to any program that receives federal assistance.

---

*In this case, Judge Rutledge states: "The law's emphasis ordinarily is on liability, not immunity, for wrongdoing. . . . Charity is generally no defense. When it has been organized as a trust or corporation, emphasis has shifted from liability to immunity. The conditions of law and of fact which created the shift have changed. The rule of immunity is out of step with the general trend of legislative and judicial policy in distributing losses incurred by individuals through the operation of an enterprise among all who benefit by it rather than in leaving them wholly to be borne by those who sustain them. The rule of immunity itself has given way gradually but steadily through widening, though not too well or consistently reasoned, modifications. It is disintegrating. . . .

"To offset the expense will be the gains of eliminating another area of what has been called 'protected negligence' and the anomaly that the institutional doer of good asks exemption from responsibility for its wrong, though all others must pay. The incorporated charity should respond as do private individuals, business corporations and others, when it does good in a wrong way."[24]

LIABILITY OF NURSES

In either event, whether the nurse alone is liable in a suit for damages as a result of some negligent act or whether both she and her employer are jointly liable, the fact that the nurse is personally liable is of serious consequence in terms of time and money. A recent Washington case illustrates this point, for there the litigation covered a period of eight years, during which time the persons were at court on numerous occasions before the injured person voluntarily dropped the charges against the student nurse in an action against her and a charitable institution.[38] That such protracted litigation is quite expensive in terms of time and money is readily apparent.

LIABILITY OF GOVERNMENT OR PUBLIC HOSPITALS

Before concluding this discussion of legal status, another situation that should be mentioned is the nurse's employment in government establishments. An increasing number of nurses enter this growing field. The question arises, "What liability falls on the government or public hospital in the various situations involving wrongs of their employees, such as nurses?" The usual answer is, "None at all." In our country, the United States and the different states cannot be sued without their consent. The general rule also supports the view that the maintenance of a hospital by a local unit of government is a governmental function. By contrast, employees of state or local government hospitals have to answer any charge of negligence and to pay damages to the patient if the suit is decided against them. In the case of the Federal Government, the Federal Torts Claims Act of 1945, with the exception of certain classes of claims specifically enumerated, confers a general waiver of Government immunity from suit for wrongs arising from the negligence of Federal Government employees.[39]

When a member of the military service dies in a U.S. hospital due to the negligence of the hospital physicians and others, the dependents cannot recover damages for wrongful death in a suit against the United States.[40] In one case, a soldier underwent surgery while in the Army. Later, when he had another operation at a Veterans' Administration hospital, a towel 30 inches long and 18 inches wide, marked "Medical Department U.S. Army," was removed from his stomach.[41] Again, the court held that the United States was not liable in damages under the F.T.C.A. for such negligence.

It was held that an Army surgeon or physician is not liable in damage for his negligence in rendering services to an enlisted soldier, who claimed that the surgeon's negligence in leaving sutures in the kidney area caused him to have a second operation and have the kidney removed.[42] While the Government does not permit recovery under the F.T.C.A., the military services do not leave those permanently injured in the line of duty uncompensated.

In a case in which the regulations did not permit the admission to the veterans hospital of a patient suffering from alcoholism, the court held that the doctor's duty does not go beyond a careful and safe delivery of the patient into competent hands.[43]

The United States has been held liable in a record judgment to an ex-sailor for negligent treatment at a Naval hospital during World War II.[44] As a part of his treatment at the Naval hospital, a radioactive substance was inserted in his nose so that x-rays could be taken. Following the treatment, the substance was not removed. The patient went to a V.A. hospital after receiving a medical discharge from the Navy, and his records were transferred. Over a period of time, he made a number of visits to the hospital, but he was not told of any danger from the substance in his nose. Eventually, when the patient had a tooth extracted, a biopsy of the material surrounding it revealed that cancer had developed from the radioactive substance irritating a pre-existing malformation in the nose. Radical surgery for the condition was carried out, causing disfigurement. The award of $725,000 was settled for $200,000 less, and thus an appeal was barred.

Another large malpractice award was received by an Army veteran who was paralyzed after he had lung surgery at a V.A. hospital.[45] During his military service, the veteran had contracted tuberculosis, for which surgery was advised. Near the conclusion of surgery, a resident, to control some bleeding, placed Oxycel gauze in the region of the intervertebral foramen, which caused spinal canal obstruction and paralysis.

The United States has been held liable in damages to minor children orphaned by the slaying of their mother when an Air Force psychiatrist was negligent and did not inform his successor of violent threats made by the airman in regard to his wife.[46] Without this information, the new psychiatrist had the airman released from the hospital after a few days; his duty assignment gave him access to weapons, one of which he used to kill his wife.

The United States has been held liable in damages to a veteran for the partial paralysis of his leg which occurred as a result of excessive pressure exerted by a defective tourniquet during surgery at a V.A. hospital.[47] During the procedure, the orderly continued for some minutes to pump air into a pneumatic tourniquet applied to the patient's thigh before he told the surgeon that the pressure gauge was not working on the cuff. Use of obviously defective equipment renders the employee and employer liable for the negligence.

Negligent use of proper equipment also renders the person liable. A retired Marine Corps sergeant received a $60,000 award against the United States for loss of visual acuity classified as industrial blindness in the injured eye due to a Navy physician's negligence in placing a heated tonometer on the patient's eyeball.[48]

However, a patient who is injured during the course of his hospitalization is not necessarily entitled to damages. During a grand mal epileptic seizure, a patient in a V.A. hospital fell from his bed and fractured his hip. Since he had been ambulatory on the day of the fall, the side rails on his bed had been removed. Considering all the circumstances, the court held he was not entitled to legal relief.[49]

When a patient in a Government hospital is injured while performing work for the hospital, he can sue and recover under the F.T.C.A. rather than accept the compensation provided by the Federal Employee's Compensation Act.[50] A patient at a U.S. Public Health Service hospital who was injured while working at a pants-pressing machine claimed that the Government was negligent in not keeping it properly repaired.

Employees in Government hospitals must consider carefully their responsibility for the care of dependents of military personnel. The standard of care required everywhere is reasonable care in accordance with the patient's apparent physical needs. Nurses in Government hospitals should not relax in their professional practice, supposing that no one can sue them or their employer. Pursuant to enabling legislation, the U.S. Government and many political subdivisions permit lawsuits. In one case, parents who brought suit on behalf of their infant daughter for injuries resulting in permanent blindness, allegedly due to the negligent use of forceps by an Air Force physician at a base hospital at the time of her delivery, were awarded $100,000 damages.[51] Likewise, in the case of a little girl born prematurely at a U.S. Naval hospital who contracted osteomyelitis and was seriously deformed thereby, the court held that the Government was negligent in permitting an inexperienced nurse, who had worked in a hospital where there were sick children, to work in a premature babies' nursery without giving her a physical examination, including a throat culture, and that such negligence had resulted in transmitting hospital staphylococcus to the baby.[52] However, in another case, in which a nurse administered intramuscular injections in each buttock of an infant at an Army hospital and the child later sustained a weakening in the right leg and foot drop which required extensive treatment, the lawsuit brought by the parents, who claimed that the injection by the nurse was done negligently so as to injure the sciatic nerve, failed.[53]

Nurses and all other employees in the Government service should give careful consideration to the effect of false statements of ex-veterans. It has been held that a nurse who was an ex-veteran will be denied the benefits of the Veterans' Preference Act if she ever denied being a veteran.[54]

Immunity of States and Subdivisions

A state government cannot be sued without its consent. The admission of liability of a state for the negligence or wrongful act of its employees or agents is comparatively recent. Three states, Illinois, Michigan and New York, now have a court of claims to handle such suits. In the remaining states, a few have a constitutional provision barring recovery against the state; a number by statute permit certain suits under specified conditions against the state; but most of the other states have not legislated on the subject.

In our American form of government, county, township, borough, municipal and village governments are subdivisions of the state created by law. Generally, in the absence of a specific law, such units are not liable for damages arising from the negligent performance of a governmental function. According to the weight of authority, in maintaining a hospital a jurisdiction is performing a governmental function. Accordingly, recovery was denied against a city hospital, because of an error of a nurse, for an unauthorized autopsy.[55] In some states, whether or not the patient pays for his services determines the question as to a hospital's being operated in a governmental or proprietary capacity. For example, when a county hospital accepted patients who were able to pay for hospitalization, it was held liable for damages caused by negligence.[56]

A county which operates a hospital for paying and nonpaying patients has been held liable to a private patient paying the usual charges who sustained severe burns when an employee negligently and carelessly placed a bedpan of boiling water under her.[57] In other states, the rule is not changed because the patient in a county or city hospital pays for his services. Thus, a Texas case held the city government was not liable for injury to a patient through negligence of a student nurse employed by the hospital. In its opinion, the court said:

> The city's maintenance of the hospital for purposes of conserving public health, receiving indigent patients, and applying money receipts to expenses, is the exercise of a governmental power so that the city is not liable for hospital employee's negligence resulting in injury to patients.[58]

A California court did not hold the county hospital responsible for injuries sustained when a delirious patient was left unattended for a short time.[59] However, the nurse was held liable for her act of negligence.

In cases involving private hospitals, whether such a hospital as well as the employee is liable for damages for injuries resulting from an act of a hospital employee depends on whether the employee exercised ordinary care at the time that the injury occurred.[60] It has been held that a private hospital is under a duty to furnish competent nurses.[61] The question of whether a nurse is an employee or not and as to what constitutes ordinary reasonable care under the circumstances has been previously discussed.

MALPRACTICE INSURANCE

It is well for the nurse employed in a Government hospital as well as in a non-Government hospital to realize that the consistent practice of her profession in the proper manner is her strongest safeguard against suits for damages. In addition, she is reminded that she may carry malpractice insurance for her personal protection. The cost of such malpractice insurance, particularly when obtained through the American Nurses' Association, is modest. In an era when the number of lawsuits against hospitals, physicians and nurses is increasing markedly, this type of insurance protection seems desirable. Such insurance provides three benefits to the policy holder: (1) in the event of an award of damages against the nurse, the insurance pays any sum within the specified limits of the policy, (2) it pays the cost of the lawyer furnished to defend the nurse who is sued in a civil court for some alleged injury resulting from her professional work, and (3) it will pay for bond for a nurse in the event it is required during an appeal. Not all lawsuits involving nurses as one of the parties result in an award against the nurse, but as Grace Barbee, lawyer for the California Nurses' Association, so aptly remarked:

It can be expensive to prove your innocence.

Many nurses work under the impression that they are protected by the hospital's insurance policy. Before relying exclusively on such insurance coverage, the prudent nurse should examine a copy of such an insurance policy and be certain of the extent of her coverage and whether or not such insurance simply protects her interests to the extent it is necessary to do so in the course of protecting the hospital's interests.

As the American Association of Industrial Nurses points out, a nurse's best and proven protection is professional competence, reinforced by a specific understanding of her responsibilities in her position. Professional liability insurance offers her additional protection. While it is possible for a company to secure a liability policy which provides individual protection for employees specifically named in it, in actual practice this is not frequently done.[62]

At least one attorney who works in the field considers professional liability insurance a must for every licensed nurse, and states that the amount depends upon three factors: (1) the type of nursing a particular nurse does, (2) the geographical area in which the nurse is located, and (3) the inclination of patients in the area to sue nurses.[63]

At the "California invitational"—a meeting of administrators, nurses, insurance executives and lawyers concerned with the state's increasing malpractice losses—eight major problem areas were identified: (1) suicide and "elopement," (2) anesthesia, (3) surgical cardiac arrest, (4) emergency room and nursing floor cardiac arrest, (5) qualification of surgical assistants and surgical privileges, (6) infection control, (7) maternal and neonatal injury, and (8) injection injury.[64] A three-prong attack was made on the problem: (1) in a series of regional meetings, "working guidelines" were developed and distributed to all hospitals and doctors, (2) under the direction of the state Medical Association, the development and evaluation of legislation to check such litigation was undertaken, and (3) a pilot study is being conducted in 10 hospitals to test arbitration as an alternative to litigation.

Since the Insurance Rating Board's new rates for hospital malpractice insurance have sharply increased, as illustrated by that of a California hospital, the soothing of a patient's psyche has been suggested to prevent lawsuits.[65] In-service programs aimed at minimizing lawsuits might well include instruction in administrative, environmental and psychological factors that influence the suit-prone patient as well as principles of malpractice law.

REFERENCES

1. *Restatement, Torts.* 1934, Sec. 281
2. Curry v. Bruns, 136 Neb. 74, 285 N.W. 88 (1939)
3. Clary v. Christiansen, 83 N.E. 2d 644 (Ohio Ct. of App., 1948)
4. Armstrong v. Wallace, 8 Cal. App., 2d 429, 37 P. 2d 467, motion denied in part, affirmed in part, 47 P. 2d 740 (1935)
5. Jefferson Electric Co. v. National Labor Relations Board, 102 F. 2d 949 (C.C.A. 1939)
6. Nickley v. Skemp, 206 Wis. 265, 239 N.W. 426 (1931)
7. Longuy v. La Société Française de Bienfaisance Mutuelle, 52 Cal. App. 370, 198 Pac. 1011 (1921)
8. 64 Stat. 512, 42 U.S.C.A. §§ 409, 410 (14) (1952)
9. 49 Stat. 622, 42 U.S.C. § 304 as amended (Supp. 1955)
10. 4 Schneider's Workmen's Compensation (1940 & supp. to date); Virginia Workmen's Compensation Law §§ 30-32; Wisconsin Workmen's Compensation Act § 102.44 and Table I; Texas Employer's Liability and Workmen's Compensation Insurance Laws, tit. 130, Rev. Civ. Stat. Tex., art. 8306, §§ 8-12 and Daily and Weekly Compensation Table and Table I; Pennsylvania Workmen's Compensation Act (Act of June 2, 1915-P.L. 736 as re-enacted and amended by Act of June 4, 1937-P.L. 1552, art. 3, §§ 306, 307; Pennsylvania Occupational Disease Act, art. 3 §§ 301-309
11. Denver v. Pollard, 417 P.2d 231 (Colo., 1966)
12. 35 Stat. 556, 37 Stat. 74, 39 Stat. 742, 63 Stat. 854; 5 U.S.C. §§ 751-777, 779-791, 793 (1952)
13. Pearch v. Canady, 52 Tenn. A. 343, 373 S.W. 2d 617 (1963)
14. Goodhart: Hospitals and Trained Nurses. 54 *Law Quarterly Review* 560 (1938) Gold v. Essex, C.C. [1942] 2 K. B. 293
15. *Restatement, Agency.* 1933 § 2(3); see also §§ 220, 250, 251
16. Ware v. Culp, 24 Cal. App. 2d 22, 74 P. 2d 283 (1938)

17. Williams v. Pomona Valley Hospital Assn., 21 Cal. App. 359, 131 Pac. 888 (1913)
18. Kamps v. Crown Heights Hospital, Inc., 251 App. Div. 849, 296 N.Y.S. 776, affirmed, 277 N.Y. 86 (1937)
19. 60 A.L.R. 303; Annotation on Moody v. Industrial Accident Commission, 204 Cal. 668, 269 Pac. 542 (1928)
20. Parkes v. Seasongood, 152 Fed. 583 (C.C.D.R.I. 1907)
21. Blyth v. Birmingham Waterworks Co., 11 Exchequer 781, 156 Eng. Rep. 1047 (Exchequer 1856). See also Osbourne v. Montgomery, 203 Wis. 223, 234 N.W. 372 (1931), and Charbonneau v. MacRury, 84 N.H. 501, 153 Atl. 457 (1931)
22. Valentin v. La Société Française de Bienfaisance Mutuelle de Los Angeles, 76 Cal. App. 2d 1, 172 P. 2d 359 (1946)
23. Piper v. Epstein, 326 Ill. App. 400, 62 N.E. 2d 139 (1945)
24. Hughes v. President and Directors of Georgetown College, 33 Fed. Supp. 867, affirmed 130 F (2d) 810 (D.C. Cir. 1942)
25. Porter v. Patterson and Emory University, 107 Ga. App. 64, 129 S.E. 2d 70 (1962)
26. Crowe v. Provost, 52 TN.Appeals 397, 374 S.W. 2d 645 (1963)
27. Regan, William A.: Nurse Shortage Remedies Can Be Risky. *Regan Report on Nursing Law,* 5 (8) 1, Jan., 1965
28. Cook v. John N. Norton Memorial Infirmary, 180 Ky.331, 202 S.W. 874 (1918)
29. Roosen v. Peter Bent Brigham Hospital, 235 Mass. 66, 126 N.E. 392 (1920)
30. Sessions v. Thomas Dee Memorial Hospital Assn., 94 Utah 460, 51 P. 2d 229 (1938)
31. O'Connor v. Boulder Colorado Sanitarium Assn., 105 Colo. 259, 96 P. 2d 835 (1939)
32. Scott, Austin W.: *Law of Trusts,* Vol. III. Boston, Little, Brown & Co., 1939, § 402, pp. 2148 ff.
33. Foye v. St. Francis Sanitarium and Training School for Nurses, 2 La. App. 305 (1925)
34. Taylor v. Flower Deaconess Home and Hospital, 104 Ohio St. 61, N.E. 287 (1922)
35. Ray v. Tucson Medical Center, 72 Ariz. 22, 230 P. 2d 220 (1951). See also Spencer: Ray v. Tuscon Medical Center, a Re-Appraisal of the Tort Liability of Charities. 24 *Rocky Mt. Law Review* 71 (1951). See also Haynes v. Presbyterian Hospital Assn., 241 Iowa 1269, 45 N.W. 2d 5 (1950), Malloy v. Fong, 232 P. 2d 241 (1951) reversing 37 Cal. 2d 356, 220 P. 2d 48
36. Adkins v. St. Francis Hospital of Charleston, W. Va., 143 S.E. 2d 154 (W. Va. 1965)
37. Sullivan v. Sisters of St. Francis, 374 S.W. 2d 294 (Ct. Civ. Appeals Texas, 1963)
38. Miller *et ux.* v. Mohr *et al.,* Miller *et ux.* v. Sisters of St. Francis *et al.,* 198 Wash. 619, 89 P. 2d 807, affirmed 105 P. 2d 32 (1940)
39. 60 Stat. 812; 28 U.S.C. §§ 1291, 1346, 1402, 1504, 2110, 2401, 2402, 2411, 2412, 2671-2680
40. Van Sickel v. United States, 56 Ca. R. 81, 285 F. 2d 87 (U.S. Ct. of Appeals, 9th Circ., Calif., 1960). See also Feres v. United States, 340 U.S. 135 (1950) concerning a serviceman in the United States who "while on active duty and not on furlough, sustained injury due to negligence of others in the armed forces."
41. Jefferson v. United States, 77 F. Supp. 706, aff'm. 178 F.2d 518, 71 S. Ct. 153 (1950)
42. Bailey v. E. Van Buskirk, 375 F. 2d 72, 345 Fed. Rep. 2d 298 (U.S. Ct. of Appeals, 9th Cir., 1965)
43. Murray v. United States 16 C C H Negl. Cases 522 (U.S. Ct. of Appeals, 4th Cir., 1964)
44. Schwartz v. United States, 16 C C H Neg. Cases 2d 1227 (USDC-Pa, 1964)
45. Christopher v. United States, 237 F. Supp. 787, 16A|2 3, 19A|2 557, 63A|2 1893, 82 A|2 1262 (U.S. Dist. Ct. E.D. Penna.) 1965
46. Underwood v. United States, 1A|2 222, 356 F. 2d 92 (U.S. Ct. of Appeals, 5th Cir., Ala., 1966)
47. Brown v. United States, 5 CCH Neg. Cases 2d 1086 (USDC-N.Y.) 1956
48. Owen v. United States, 251 F. Supp. 38 (1966)
49. Greenberger v. United States, 17 CCH Neg. 2d 1254 (USDC-N.Y.) 1965
50. United States v. Martinez, 334 Fed (2d) 728 (U.S. Ct. of Appeals, 10th Cir., Colo., 1964)
51. Larabee v. United States, 13 CCH Neg. 2d 1001
52. Kapuschinsky v. United States, 248 F. Supp. 732(1966)

53. Evans v. United States, 212 F. Supp. 648 (D.C. Mass., 1962), 15 CCH Neg. 2d 989
    (U.S. Ct. of Appeals, 1st Cir., 1963)
54. Vigdor v. United States Civil Service Commission, 254 Fed. 2d 333 (1958)
55. Schwab v. Connelly, 116 Colo. 195, 179 P. 2d 667 (1947)
56. Henderson v. Twin Falls County, 56 Idaho 124, 50 P. 2d 597 (1935)
57. Hernandez v. The County of Yuma, 91Az.35 369 P. 2d 271 (1962)
58. City of McAllen v. Gartmen *et ux.,* 81 S.W. 2d 147, affirmed 107 S.W. 879 (Ct. Civ.
    Appeals Tex., 1937)
59. Griffin v. County of Colusa *et al.,* 44 Cal. App. 2d 915, 113 P. 2d 270 (141)
60. Dahlberg v. Jones, 232 Wis. 6, 285 N.W. 841 (1939); Wetzel v. Omaha Maternity,
    etc., 96 Neb. 636, 148 N.W. 582 (1914)
61. Goldfoot v. Lofgren, 135 Ore. 533, 296 Pac. 843 (1931)
62. Professional Liability Information (Editorial). *Am. Assn. Indust. Nurses,* 16:23-24,
    Oct., 1968
63. Insurance: A "Must" for Every Licensed Nurse. *Regan Report on Nursing Law,* 10
    (3) 1, August, 1969
64. Foster, John T.: What California Is Doing about It. *Modern Hosp.,* 112: 84, Feb.,
    1969
65. Bernzweig, Eli P.: Soothing Patient Psyche May Prevent Lawsuit. *Modern Hosp.,*
    112: 83-86, 104, Feb., 1969

Chapter Six

The Relation of a Nurse's Rights and Liabilities to Her Position and Status

NURSES' LIABILITIES AND RIGHTS

In any occupation, the person who works and the persons for whom the work is done must "keep the law." The practice of nursing is no exception. Suits at law fall into two classes of actions: those involving a breach of contract, and those involving torts, or injuries or wrongs to the person or property of another. Those actions in which a nurse is one of the parties are frequently either suits involving disagreements over contracts for personal services or for damages for injuries as a result of negligence to the person or property of another. Situations resulting in claims for damages can be handled by a lawsuit or settlement. Laws of the different states vary considerably as to the liability that can be imposed for the injuries and wrongs done by another, for example, as an employee or agent.

LIABILITY FOR NEGLIGENCE

It is important to keep in mind that liability for negligence does not depend upon a legal relationship or a contract between the persons. A nurse who in some manner causes injury to a patient can be sued for damages by the patient, regardless of who may employ or pay the nurse or whether the services are given for pay or given gratuitously. Of course, as has been pointed out, a nurse may also be sued in some cases for breach of contract to give proper nursing care. Whether the nurse is an independent contractor, agent or employee is important in ascertaining the liability of other persons in addition to the nurse in damage suits arising from negligence. The employer's degree of control, the type of business, the basis and method of payment, the place and equipment are some factors considered in differentiating employees from independent contractors.

In some states, nurses when engaged in strictly professional duties are considered independent contractors and, as such, solely liable for their actions. In a number of states, the liability of an employer for a nurse's professional acts depends on his status, i.e., whether he is considered an employee of a governmental, private profit-making or charitable institution. Again, whether the nurse is a general duty or special duty nurse is a determining factor. On the other hand, in a few states, in an institution where a nurse engaged in an "administrative" or "ministerial" act not connected with the patient's medical care, the hospital has been held liable in damages.

Administrative or ministerial acts are those not connected with the patient's medical care. For example, making a patient's bed, or adjusting a window for air, or serving his tray, or putting side rails on his bed would be considered such an act. When a patient was left alone while under anesthesia and fell from bed and was injured because the head nurse had failed to have side rails attached to the bed, the hospital was liable because the negligence was "administrative."[1] Professional duties are those connected with a patient's nursing or medical needs. For example, when a child two years of age fell out of a crib and was injured, the hospital was not held liable in an action for damages because the negligence was professional rather than administrative. Here the determination or evaluation by the nurse of the necessity and adequacy of restraints for the child was looked upon as a professional duty.[2]

Again, in determining negligence, the nurse is reminded that we must determine it from all the circumstances.[3] The question arises whether the nurse acted as a person with average skill in her calling, placed in similar circumstances, would have acted, or whether she used less care, judgment or skill. Moreover, the nurse is cautioned to realize that it is not enough to do what is usual if the act ordinarily done is careless, because no one can claim he is not liable for failure to use due care for the reason that others are as careless as he is.

Care in Emergency Situations

The nurse should know that whatever moral or humanitarian obligations there may be, there is no obligation or duty in the absence of a statutory provision to give care to a person in an emergency.[4] For example, in some states there is a law expressly stating that a person involved in an automobile accident in which persons are injured must not leave without giving aid. However, when an obligation is undertaken voluntarily, it becomes her duty to give every necessary service that the situation calls for. For example, the court has stated that no one is obliged by law to assist a stranger, even though he can do so by a word and without the slightest danger to himself, but once he has undertaken to give assistance, the law imposes on him a duty of care toward the person assisted.[5]

Another circumstance that may affect liability or negligence is whether the act was done in an emergency situation. Under emergency circumstances, a nurse, like any other person, may perform a medical act to preserve life and limb. Either law or custom exempts such acts from coming within the medical practice acts. However, whether there is in fact an "emergency" is a question that has to be decided in view of all the circumstances. The nurse is reminded that in view of her education, training and experience, she will be held to a higher degree of care than an ordinary person who acts in an emergency. In other words, she will be expected to act like an ordinary nurse under similar circumstances.

Good Samaritan legislation is designed to encourage volunteer first aid in emergency situations. However, such statutes offer little help in determining whether or not a true emergency does exist. Since numbers of apparent emergencies are borderline situations, the decision that a real emergency exists is important for two reasons: it typically relieves the first aider of the consequences of his acts (except for willful misconduct), and certain statutory restrictions on performing medical acts are suspended for the emergency. The determination that a particular set of facts constitutes an emergency is legally correct only when it can be shown that reasonable and prudent men would have reached the same decision under the same or similar circumstances. Moreover, at the time of a trial, which is generally several years later than the accident that gave rise to it, the emergency character of many situations may seem less than at the time of occurrence. Hence, the need for a first aid person to correctly evaluate situations as to their emergency character, as judged at a later time by reasonable and prudent men, is not relieved by Good Samaritan laws and may in fact be a deterrent to their intervention.[5a]

The professional nurse in the emergency room must make rapid decisions, screen patients, have knowledge of how to assist in all types of emergency care and have the ability to deal appropriately with people under stress.[6] Both the professional nurse and her personnel must be prepared to render effective nursing care in emergencies. Consequently, they must have knowledge concerning a variety of emergencies and must keep abreast of new developments in this type of nursing. When the emergency patient arrives, emergency drugs, equipment and supplies must be on hand and in working order for immediate use.

The nurse should know that neither she nor her employer incurs tort liability unless there has been a deviation from certain standards. To specify precisely what is expected by way of nursing care is not easy. If a hospital participates in Medicare or Health Insurance for the Aged, one must know the following "Conditions for Participation":[7]

1. Standard A. Factor 3. The emergency service is supervised by a qualified member of the medical staff and the nursing functions are the responsibility of a registered professional nurse.
2. Standard C. Factor 1. The medical staff is responsible for insuring adequate medical coverage for emergency services.
3. Standard C. Factor 2. Qualified physicians are regularly available at all times for the emergency service, either day or on call.
4. Standard C. Factor 3. A physician sees all patients who arrive for treatment in the emergency service.
5. Standard C. Factor 4. Qualified nurses are available on duty at all times, and in sufficient number to deal with the number and extent of emergency services.

These provisions do cover the matter of staffing in the emergency room, which at various times has been a matter of concern. Furthermore, as Dr. Letourneau has pointed out in an article, any deviation from these standards may lead to a presumption of negligence.[8]

Many times the emergency room nurse must make decisions as to whether an emergency exists. In one case, an action for wrongful death of an infant who died shortly after treatment was refused at a private hospital which maintained an emergency ward.[9] The infant, who had a temperature and diarrhea and had not slept for two nights, was brought in by his parents, who told the nurse that the child was under the care of two doctors and showed her the medicine prescribed. The nurse explained to the parents that the hospital could not give treatment because the child was under the care of a physician and that the medicine of the hospital might conflict with that of the doctor. She did not examine the child, but tried unsuccessfully to get in touch with his doctors. She suggested that the parents bring the child to the pediatric clinic the next morning. During the night, the baby died of bronchial pneumonia. An order for summary judgment for the hospital was denied, and the court said the question was whether the nurse's determination not to have the infant examined by an intern was within reasonable limits of judgment of a graduate nurse, even though mistaken, or whether she was derelict in her duty as a graduate nurse in not recognizing an emergency from the symptoms related to her.

In a New York case, a widow sought recovery of damages for

wrongful death from a hospital and a physician for failure to render necessary emergency treatment to a patient who came to the emergency room after awakening with severe pains in his chest and arms.[10] He mentioned that they were members of the Hospital Insurance Plan (HIP). The nurse stated that the hospital had no connections with HIP and did not take care of HIP patients. The nurse did call a HIP doctor, and let the patient describe his complaints to him. The doctor told him to go home and return when HIP was open. After that, the nurse refused to summon another doctor to examine the man. Thereafter, the man and his wife returned home, where he died before help could be secured. The New York Supreme Court reversed the trial court's verdict for the hospital and said that there was a question whether the physician who talked to the decedent and whether the hospital's nurse who allegedly refused to have the decedent examined, were negligent.

In still another case, in which a patient with a myocardial infarct was brought to the emergency room and examined by the nurses, they decided there was no emergency and a physician was not called.[11] Later, he was examined by a physician, who had him admitted to the hospital as an emergency patient, and he died two days later. The nurses erred in making a decision that was not theirs to make. However, the hospital was not held liable, since physicians testified that the delay in admitting the patient made no difference in his death.

Every professional nurse in the emergency room should know the standards for the emergency department published by the American College of Surgeons, which states:

> The function of an emergency department is to give adequate appraisal and initial treatment or advice to every person who considers himself acutely ill or injured and presents himself at the emergency department door.[12]

Since many emergency rooms are clogged with patients with assorted minor ailments, and it appears that many come in the evenings because they find emergency room hours more convenient than clinic hours, it seems necessary to point out to the professional nurse the necessity of establishing some system of priorities such as that of triage. Otherwise, if a "first come, first served" basis is used, a person with a severe myocardial infarction or a depressed skull fracture might have to wait for long periods in the emergency room while physicians examined numbers of patient with common colds, minor cuts, sprains and so forth; and such a scheme scarcely meets the standard of what an ordinary, reasonable and prudent person would do as is required by the law.

The professional nurse in the emergency room must realize that only complete and accurate emergency room records will adequately serve the needs of the patient, the physician, the emergency room staff and the hospital for medico-legal purposes.[13]

A nurse should pursue her profession to the best of her ability and understanding, remembering that she is responsible for her own negligence and torts. The previous chapter discussed the effect which the type of institution in which a nurse may work—governmental, private, or charitable—may have upon employer's liability for negligence or wrongful acts of employees. Moreover, a nurse in her contracts for service, like every other person, is governed by the law of contracts. To avoid liability on her personal service contracts, she must do none of the inexcusable acts noted in Chapter IV.

PROFESSIONAL REGISTERED NURSE'S LEGAL STATUS

By way of clarifying a nurse's legal status, professional registered nurses may be grouped into two classes based upon the type of work performed, as suggested by the American Nurses' Association.[14] The first group consists of those nurses in the actual practice of nursing, as done by the general duty nurse, private duty nurse, public health staff nurse, school nurse, industrial nurse and office nurse. It is true that in some instances such nurses may have additional duties, but in the aggregate this group consists of persons who are not only nurses, but also persons who give nursing care to individual patients. A second group consists of persons who are primarily concerned with other aspects of nursing which further the patient's care and welfare by handling the requisite administrative, educational and supervisory matters related to such service, such as supervision, administration, consultation and teaching. These persons as a group do not themselves usually give individual care to the patient, but through their work prepare and assist other nurses to do so, or further the patient's care and welfare by handling necessary administrative and supervisory matters connected with it.

Though it has been pointed out that there are nurse practice acts in every state which outline precisely what a nurse may do, her duties are not defined or set forth except in general terms. However, it is evident that a nurse must not do any act that might be interpreted as the practice of medicine;[15] and the nurse's acts, aside from emergency situations, must be performed under the direction or supervision of a licensed physician.[16] From the decided cases, it appears that a licensed nurse may do all those professional acts which she is ordinarily and customarily taught to do and does do in schools of nursing which are approved by the jurisdiction, if the acts are done to a patient in accordance with the direction and supervision of his physician.

There is a conflict of authority and opinion on the question of whether or not a nurse is protected when she acts upon the orders of an unlicensed physician, such as an intern. On the whole, interns are not licensed to practice medicine, although, as in New York, they may be expressly allowed to practice medicine within a hospital.[17] Whether an intern or resident is the agent of the patient's physician depends on whether or not the physician has the right to direct not only the work to be done, but also the details of doing it. If the intern is an agent of a licensed physician acting within the scope of his employment when giving orders to the nurse, the nurse is protected. In any event, it would seem advisable for a nurse to know the legal status of an intern in the particular jurisdiction in which she works.

Nurses must obey the orders of the physician in charge of a patient, unless an order is such as to lead a reasonable person to anticipate injury if it were carried out.[18] However, this does not mean that a nurse can go ahead and willy-nilly unquestioningly carry out the doctor's orders. For example, in a case in which a nurse was giving a hypodermoclysis and noticed that the patient was not properly absorbing the fluid, since she neither discontinued it nor called a doctor, she was held liable for negligence.[19] On going to a hospital, a physician has the right to assume, in the absence of contrary information, that the nurses in the hospital not directly employed by him or working directly under him are competent.[20]

Telephone Orders

Telephone orders constitute a real problem for nurses in a number of situations. The best interests of the patient, physician, nurse and hospital or other agency are served by having all orders of the physician in writing. When a physician telephones an order, he should sign in on his next visit. The nurse accepting the telephoned order should read it back to the physician to make certain she has correctly written down the order. Concerning who may accept telephone orders, Emanual Hayt stated some years ago:

> Telephone orders may be given to the director of nurses, any resident or intern, the night supervisor, a floor supervisor, senior nurse or a private duty nurse.[21]

Adherence to this recommended policy is desirable. There is no question that it strictly limits the number of nurses accepting telephone orders, and in the interest of safety this is desirable. Granted, anyone can make an error, but studies show that fewer errors are made by those who have more education, including a greater knowledge of drugs. The person who takes the telephone order should sign the name of the physician *per* her own name. However, if the nurse has any question about the suitability of such an order in view of the patient's apparent condition, she should ask a resident physician to examine the order to check that it is not inconsistent with the patient's needs. When a problem appears, the order should be verified with the prescribing physician.

True, in an emergency the telephone order may be the only way to secure needed medical advice. In such situations, as in the case of an ill seaman on a ship without a physician, telephone orders are necessary and the court will uphold those who act upon them.[22] Nevertheless, nurses and doctors should limit telephone orders to true emergency situations in which there is no alternative, since the use of a telephone in a nonemergency situation as a substitute for the physician himself actually seeing and evaluating the patient can lead to serious error and may border on malpractice.[23]

The California Appellate Court has held that an identification based on a "voice print" was improperly admitted in evidence. The "voice print" technique is not generally accepted at present by the scientific community.[24]

Transcribing Orders

In many hospitals today, ward secretaries or clerks transcribe orders. It is important that they be thoroughly instructed in transcribing the order as it is written by the physician. Moreover, the ward secretary or clerk should know that she is liable for her own errors, for at law everyone is liable for his own errors and can be sued for damages for negligence. The requirement that the transcribed order must be countersigned by a professional registered nurse is common. If the nurse countersigns an order incorrectly transcribed by the ward secretary or clerk, she is liable for her error. However, if the nurse also errs, this does not relieve the ward secretary or clerk for her own error. If two persons both made an error, both can be sued; and in addition, if they are employees of a hospital or other agency, then pursuant to the doctrine of *respondeat superior,* it, too, can be sued.

PHYSICIANS' ASSISTANTS

Due to the shortage of physicians in our country and the rising demand for their services, a few universities have made innovations in the training of paramedical personnel. One such program to emerge has been that of preparing physicians' assistants to work with the doctor. Currently, such an individual is not licensed as a physician's assistant, but receives a certificate from the educational institution at the completion of his two-year educational period. His duties are determined by the physician to whom he is responsible and include history-taking, portions of physical examinations, assorted technical procedures, and instruction of and reassurance of patients — to mention a few items. While present laws permit dependent functions of assistants within defined classes such as nurses, physical therapists and laboratory technicians, state medical practice acts must be changed to permit new categories while protecting the public from poorly trained assistants and poorly conceived and planned experimental educational programs. The reader desiring more information concerning this new category of paramedical worker will find references at the end of this chapter.[25] The suggestion has also been made that if physicians analyzed how they deliver health care, they would find that they could turn over additional major portions of their work to nurses.[26] While legally this may be true, the desirability thereof is another matter, since there is a shortage of professional nurses, too.

PERSONAL LIABILITY IN CIVIL ACTION FOR NEGLIGENCE

A nurse should remember that she is liable for her own negligent acts. Consequently, if she carelessly injures her patient's property, such as his personal belongings, she may incur liability. When a patient wearing two rings was operated on in a hospital and, while she was unconscious, one ring disappeared, although the surgeons and nurses present said they did not know what became of it, the private hospital was held liable. The patient said that on admission she was asked only to surrender her money for safekeeping; however, there was a duty to protect her other property while she was helpless.[27] The court stated that the liability of the hospital for its employees, nurses and physicians was like that of a railroad or steamship company to passengers for the acts of its employees. Also, a hospital has been held liable when a patient sued for damages for loss of his bridgework through the negligence of a nurse.[28]

When a patient dies, the nurse should know that the property of the deceased may be given only to the legal representative of the estate upon his producing a certified copy of his appointment as executor or administrator. As a practical proposition, considering the risks involved, articles of little or no value may be turned over to the decedent's family or next of kin and a signed receipt therefor obtained. However, in the case of valuables, if the nurse is involved, she should realize the risk in any failure to observe the law.

As has been previously discussed, supervisors may be held liable for the actions of others under certain circumstances.

In this chapter, attention is focused upon the theories underlying legal liability of the nurse for damages arising out of her acts. There is no one set of factors that will decide the legal status of a nurse in a lawsuit. The decision in each case is governed by the facts in the particular case. However, some matters that the court tries to ascertain in order to establish a nurse's legal status are whether she is an employee or independent contractor and what is the degree of control retained or given up by the nurse. As pointed out in a previous chapter, this is determined by examining the contract. As the majority of contracts for nursing service are implied contracts, testimony and evidence may be necessary to show the real relationship between the persons.

In the eyes of the law, the licensed nurse's work is based on skills acquired through education and training. A typical statute is that of Maine, which expresses her status as follows:

> The registration and certification of professional trained nurses is to designate by public registry and certification those nurses for whose qualifications the state is willing to vouch, and to prevent others who are not entitled to it from falsely claiming such sponsorship.[29]

The nurse is personally liable in a civil action if a patient is injured because of incompetence or carelessness in the performance of her skills and duties. If her negligent acts show a wanton and reckless conduct or disregard for human life, such a degree of negligence is considered "gross negligence," which the law views as criminal. Reference to specific skills and duties will aid in spelling out the degree of care and prudence demanded by the law.

Importance of Proper Records and Charts

In regard to charts, nurses have important responsibilities. On each sheet of the chart, the name of the patient and date should be properly filled in for identification. Since erasures in records may create suspicion as to the reason for the change, it would be preferable practice to make none, but rather to draw one line through the incorrect matter, add the date and signature of the person doing so, and then add the correct material. As one writer has pointed out in discussing hospital records, the charts of every hospital should be kept so as to show that consent to surgery was given by the patient preceding the administration of narcotics or sedatives.[30] Otherwise, as in a California case, if a patient has not signed such consent prior to receiving sedatives and narcotics, the reality of consent may be effectively questioned. Since the nurse is the person who customarily attends to securing the patient's signature on the form giving consent for surgery, she should be aware of this point.

The California Hospital Association publishes a Consent Manual which is brought up to date every two years. A consent is valid in the hospital for a reasonable period of time.

In negligence actions against doctors, nurses and hospitals the nurse should realize the value of complete charting. For example, when it is customary for a physician to visit his hospital patients each morning, consider the effect in a malpractice action of a nurse's chart which did not record his visits for four or five days at a time. Again, for her own protection, a nurse should chart routine procedures. For example, if a nurse is being questioned as to why the chart does not show that she checked the color of the patient in the parts affected by a cast, it is discouraging to her defense when she says, "Oh, I know I did it; I always do; that's why I don't chart it."

At least in California, new court decisions will require more accurate and circumspect record keeping, since any patient has the right to obtain hospital medical records on request.[31]

Accurate, truthful nurses' notes, which record what the nurse has observed and heard first-hand, are of great value. In the search for the truth in regard to an accident in the hospital, the hour-by-hour record made by on-the-scene nurses of what transpired is carefully reviewed. On the whole, it is probably the best evidence we may have of the true situation. In some instances, the patient's lack of obedience to doctor's orders may indicate contributory negligence, while in other instances his repeated complaints warn of problems before it is "too late" to avoid deleterious consequences. Considerable care must be used in streamlining the nurses' charting to insure that we continue to adequately discharge the nurses' function of recording and reporting, for a series of predetermined signs and symbols does not always accurately reflect all of the pertinent observations of the patient's condition, let alone the nurse's evaluation thereof or her plan of nursing care.

In a recent case, the appellate court ruled that the trial court committed serious error in not admitting to evidence the nurse's notes.[32] The plaintiff obtained an award for $4500 in a malpractice suit, but the nurse's notes on the plaintiff's chart for the days in question indicated that he slept well, was up and around as he chose and made no complaints, so it was prejudicial to exclude them. Although nurses' notes on a chart are bulky and storage of medical records requires valuable space, they should be preserved at least for the statutory period in which a suit could be brought against the hospital, personnel and doctors, and the need for micro-filming them, or at least for doing so with selected records, warrants careful consideration.

The use of ward secretaries and clerks to transcribe doctors' orders in many hospitals today is not without its problems and errors. The ward secretary or clerk who transcribes the doctor's order to a Kardex or other type of record should know and appreciate that she is personally liable (in addition to her employer) for any errors she may make in so doing. Moreover, the nurse who countersigns the transcribed orders or requisitions is responsible for her own action.

The case of *Engle v. Clarke* et al. deserves mention for the excellence of the nurses' charting and nursing care.[33] The patient had undergone surgery to correct an epigastric hernia, and after a downward postoperative course he died and a malpractice suit was brought against the doctor. In finding for the doctor, the court said:

> The patient did not have a special nurse but received excellent attention from hospital personnel. At 3 P.M. he was nauseated and was given Dramamine. At 4 P.M. Mrs. McReynolds, the supervising nurse on duty from 3–11 P.M. was concerned over his progress. He was cold, clammy, pale, restless, and sweating profusely. McReynolds telephoned Dr. Scott at his office. He instructed her to go ahead and give the patient a medication (Dramamine) and said he probably would come to the hospital later in the afternoon. Glucose was administered at this time, and blood pressure stood at 120/80. The patient was nauseated at 5 P.M. and at 6 P.M. his color was still more pallid; he was cold, in an anxious state, and there was a 10-point downward change in blood pressure. . . .

The entire record, only a portion of which is quoted, reflects good nurses' charting which greatly aided the court in its search for true facts.

On the other hand, in another lawsuit against the state for damages following the death of a mentally ill girl, the chart showed that the patient's temperature was 101.8° on March 13 and 104° on March 16, without any effort at treatment or any nurses' notes for March 14 and 15. It was held to be evidence of the hospital's lack of ordinary and reasonable care of the patient.[34]

Several recent California decisions have upheld the right of any patient to obtain hospital medical records on request.[35] Nurses as well as physicians and hospitals will have to adapt to this change.

Gabriel has pointed out that the following medico-legal cases may need reference to the nurses' notes or observations: (1) personal injury cases, such as traffic victims, (2) insurance cases when patients try to collect, (3) workmen's compensation cases, (4) will probates in which nurses' notes may show the condition of the patient with respect to consciousness or testamentary capacity, and (5) criminal cases.[36] In order to avoid lawsuits and charges of negligence, the nurses' charting on such patients must be complete and pertinent.

Incident Report

An incident report or unusual occurrence form[37] was designed to serve four functions: (1) improving the management and treatment of the patient, (2) in-service education of residents, nurses and others, (3) administrative supervision, and (4) medico-legal coverage. By careful wording, chosen to avoid the implication of blame and retribution, by routing it through key members of the teaching and administrative staff and by classifying the incident for statistical tabulation, the form provided for these requirements.

Criminal Liability for Negligence

If a patient is injured by an unavoidable accident, such as one resulting from an intervening force of nature while he is in the care of a nurse, she will not be liable.[38] However, if the accident could have been avoided by the ordinary use of her skills and prudence, she may be held liable.

DEFENSE IN COURT ACTIONS FOR NEGLIGENCE

It is instructive to consider the defenses a nurse may have to actions for damages due to injuries caused by negligence.

Idiosyncrasy

Generally, a claim of idiosyncrasy (peculiarity of constitution) of the patient can be a defense to negligence. The meaning of this claim is that the patient had some peculiarity which made him unusually susceptible to a treatment or drug which in normal persons would be reasonably safe, and that the peculiarity was of such a kind that the nurse, using average care and skill, could not have discovered it. For example, when a patient who received x-ray treatment sued for damages for burns, the court said that a patient receiving x-ray treatment assumes the risk of burn from proper treatment, but the physician incurs liability for causing negligent burns.[39] The same result would be true if the defendant were a nurse. However, by express provision of law, the defense that one has assumed the risk is done away with in cases coming within the Workmen's Compensation Laws.

Remoteness of Cause of Injury

Again, the nurse might claim remoteness of cause of injury as a defense. For a negligence to be actionable, the breach of duty must be the "proximate cause of injury"; that is, one that in the usual course of events would not happen in lieu of the cause. For example, suppose a patient who was incapable of using sound judgment was placed in a sanitarium; assume further that one day the patient wandered away and onto a railroad track where a train struck and killed him, whereupon the patient's executor brought an action for damages against the head nurse on the floor in the sanitarium from which the patient wandered away. In such a case the negligent acts of the head nurse were not the proximate cause of death, but only a condition which made a fatal injury possible.[40]

Contributory Negligence

A frequent defense interposed is that of contributory negligence. Contributory negligence is used to describe any unreasonable conduct on the part of the patient which is the cause of injury, whether the nurse is also negligent or not. For example, suppose a patient sued a nurse for damages due to burns caused by negligently applying an electric heating pad. Assume further that the evidence showed that the patient's physician had ordered hot moist packs and the use of an electric heating pad to keep the packs hot. The evidence, moreover, showed that the patient had control over the switch to the electric heating pad and that he used it without difficulty for four days, but later went to sleep with the switch on and suffered some burns. Since the patient's negligence contributed to his injury, the case against the nurse would be dismissed.[41]

In a case in which a nurse's aide emerged from a utility room without looking into the corridor and sustained injuries when she collided with a delivery man carrying a vase of flowers, she was denied recovery in a lawsuit because she was guilty of contributory negligence.[42] The court said:

> As a nurse's aide, aware of the use of the corridor for disabled patients in wheelchairs, nurses, doctors, delivery men and the like, she had a duty to determine before emerging from the door whether there was anyone in the corridor with whom she would collide.

When the parents of a deceased 2½-year-old child brought a malpractice action against the doctor for damages for wrongful death of the child in his office, and the physician alleged the contributory negligence of the parents in caring for the child, the jury exonerated the physician.[43] The child was brought to the doctor with a boil on her left shoulder. He administered penicillin and ordered hot packs applied every three to four hours and a check on the child's temperature with a baby fever thermometer. The hot packs were not applied as ordered, as the child spent time with each of the parents (who were separated), the temperature was taken with an ordinary oral thermometer and the child allowed to play outside. An autopsy showed anaphylaxis due to Xylocaine used before opening the boil and to toxemia due to bacteria from the abscess.

Judgment was entered for the defendant doctor in a suit brought by a patient for damages for ruptured ear drums in which he was contributorily negligent in insisting that the nurse wash the wax from his ears.[44]

However, the nurse is reminded that by express provision of law, the defense of contributory negligence is done away with in cases coming within the Workmen's Compensation Laws.

Statute of Limitations

The statute of limitations as a defense to an action to recover damages for negligence has already been discussed.

Release Agreement

There is an old maxim to the effect that one who consents to an act *prima facie* (on first appearance) wrongful cannot afterward complain of it. However, it is pointed out that contracts which "contract out" liability for negligence are looked upon with disfavor by the law. In some jurisdictions, one cannot avoid liability for negligence by contract.[45] In any jurisdiction, such a contract would be strictly interpreted against the person claiming it as a defense. However, the nurse is reminded that a contract for indemnity from such liability is valid.

Sometimes a release may be a good defense against an action for damages for injuries caused by negligence. For example, in the case of a physician, the release of an automobile driver from liability for injury to a patient struck by the automobile driver barred the patient's action against the physician for negligence in caring for the injury because damages for the same could have been gotten from the automobile driver.[46] Or again, suppose that a nurse agrees to give up her right to compensation, in return for which a patient agrees to release her from possible legal action. The nurse could use such an agreement as a defense in any action the patient might bring later.

Registered nurses are reminded that they are professional people and that their status has been elevated in recent years. As a consequence, nurses' earnings have increased, and this may give a new direction to damage suits. Perhaps in bygone years the patient did not think it worthwhile to seek damages from nurses on account of their mistakes. Today this viewpoint is changing. Nurses who make mistakes or are careless cannot depend on being "let off," but will have to face their responsibility.[47]

MASTER-SERVANT RELATIONSHIPS

General Duty Nurse in Hospital

The general duty nurse usually performs her duties as an employee of the hospital or institution that engages her services.[48] The contract does not indicate a nurse-patient relationship; but the nurse's wages are paid by the employer, who furnishes her place of employment and necessary working equipment, and the nurse's services are carried out in relation to the general business of the employer. It is generally considered that the hospital-employer not only controls the work to be done, but also has authority to supervise and regulate the means by which it is done.

General Duty Nurse to Physician or Patient

When a hospital assigns a general duty nurse to a physician or a patient, the nurse is in a different status. She is no longer a general duty nurse in the hospital, but an employee of the physician or a special duty nurse of the patient. For example, a court has held that when a hospital nurse was under the operating surgeon's special supervision and control during an operation upon a patient, although she was not in his regular employment, the relationship of master and servant existed.[49] In another case, a patient who sustained a fractured rib as a result of a nurse's applying pressure to her body during delivery was denied recovery in a lawsuit against the hospital.[50] The Vermont Supreme Court held that the doctor, who was not selected nor employed by the hospital, had complete control and supervision of the nurses in the delivery room, and that the hospital therefore was not responsible for the negligent performance of the nurse in carrying out his order. However, in the absence of a specific contract, a physician is not responsible for the negligent acts of a nurse in treating a patient after the operation unless he undertakes to continue his control of the nurse.[51]

However, in New York, the nurse, in doing routine duties such as giving a bedpan, is an employee or servant of the hospital. But when the nurse is carrying out her professional acts concerned with the patient's medical or nursing needs, i.e., following the physician's orders, the nurse may be an independent contractor.[52] Sometimes the question of the relationship between the parties becomes a question of fact for the jury to decide. The general duty nurse's functions (including those of a head nurse) are outlined in descriptive statements developed by the American Nurses' Association.[53]

Liability of Employer

When the general duty nurse is considered an employee, whether, in addition to herself, her employer is liable in damages for her acts may be governed by whether the employer is a governmental, charitable or profit-making institution. For example, when a nurse was lowering a hospital bed by mechanical means and did not warn the patient of the hazards, which inflicted injury to his fingers, so that they later had to be amputated, the hospital was held liable for the nurse's carelessness.[54]

In an era of nurse shortage, employers should bear in mind that from the legal standpoint there must be sufficient nurse coverage to meet the apparent needs of the patients. To meet hospital needs, nurses from overseas as well as from within the United States have been recruited. Greater use of practical nurses, nurses prepared in associate degree programs and nursing students (who work for pay outside school hours) has followed. The inactive nurse has been encouraged to return to work and in some instances refresher courses have been provided to facilitate her return to active duty. It is important for directors of nursing, hospital administrators, nursing home administrators and others to realize that the doctrine of *respondeat superior* applies to all employees.[55]

Private Duty Nurse

In the ordinary case, the law looks upon the private duty nurse (special duty nurse) as an independent contractor. It is the intention of the parties that the nurse shall not be under the control of the patient as to the details of the nursing services. The American Nurses' Association defines the private duty nurse as follows:

> A private duty nurse is a registered professional nurse who independently contracts to give expert bedside nursing care to one patient. This permits the nurse to utilize professional knowledge and skills to the fullest extent and to assume responsibility for the total nursing care of the patient.[56]

Among the more important functions in her supervision of the patient, she is expected to plan the care, to observe, evaluate and report symptoms and reactions of the patient, to carry out independent nursing procedures, and also to perform treatments under the direction or supervision of a licensed physician. It is important for her to keep adequate and accurate records for the benefit of the patient and all medical and nursing personnel connected with his care.

The private duty nurse has a right to sue a patient if he fails to pay her wages or if he wrongfully discharges her in violation of the terms of the employment contract. The private duty nurse is also liable to the patient for any breach of contract or any wrongs or acts of negligence.

Although the private duty nurse is an independent contractor, the supervising nurse in a hospital may give her advice from time to time in regard to her patient. Though the private duty nurse and her patient must comply with the hospital's rules and regulations if they wish to use its facilities, the hospital has no right to dismiss such a nurse or to take her from her patient and reassign her to the care of others.[57] The acts of a private duty nurse do not make the hospital liable, since she is not an employee, nor subject to its control.[58] When a person wrongfully interferes with a private duty nurse's right to work in a hospital or institution, he is liable in an action for damages based thereon.[59] A private duty nurse is entitled to damages for injuries caused by the negligence of a hospital, its employees, servants or agents.[60]

As long as the private duty nurse is elected and paid by the patient, family or doctor, there was no question about her status as an independent contractor. Now that private duty nurses are usually obtained from a nurses' registry and the hospital may insist its approval be obtained for anyone who is allowed to care for a patient in it or that she be under the supervision of the hospital's nursing supervisor, she may be regarded as an employee of the hospital. In *Emory University v. Shadburn,* in which the hospital selected the private duty nurse, received payment for her services and later settled with her, the hospital was held liable for her negligence.[61] If the trend toward hospitals' responsibility for all nursing care becomes the general rule, then her status is likely to change. To date, she has generally been denied the benefits of workmen's compensation when injured on duty in the hospital.[62]

A 65-year-old licensed practical nurse coming to work who was injured in a fall on the icy sidewalk outside a nursing home was denied a recovery of damages. Although the defendant nursing home had the duty to exercise ordinary care to keep the premises in a reasonably safe condition and to give warning of any hidden defects, so as not to expose the nurse to unnecessary danger, both nurse and nursing home had knowledge of the freezing and icy conditions.[63]

A practical nurse injured her back in a hospital while helping an elderly patient from a whirlpool bath. This injury prevented her from performing heavy tasks and she was awarded workmen's compensation benefits of $28.61 a week for total disability.[64] The order was affirmed on appeal.

When an experienced practical private nurse was hurt while attending to a patient in a wheelchair in a Maryland nursing home, she was held not to be an employee and not entitled to recover workmen's compensation.[65] The court pointed out:

> The most important and really decisive common law test is whether there is a right to control and direct the worker in the performance and manner of doing his work.

It also listed some other criteria, such as selection and engagement of the worker, power of dismissal, and payment of wages. In conclusion, the court said that the private duty nurse was not an employee of the home.

Public Health Staff Nurse and School Nurse
Employees

The public health staff nurse and the school nurse have a similar status and will be discussed together. Generally, such a nurse is an employee of a department of health, board of education or voluntary agency. In order to carry out or complete the contract for rendering nursing service, the principal who is legally responsible for the same must, as a practical necessity, get an agent or agents to carry out the details. As previously discussed, the relationship between principal and agent makes the principal liable for the acts of his agent when acting within the scope of his employment. The people of the community represented by the board of health or education may be regarded as the principal, while the health officer, nurses and other employees may be considered the agents thereof. In cases in which the courts have held that the authority for appointing the health officer was the same as for appointing nurses and other employees, he was held to be an employee under the direction, supervision and control of the board of health.[66]

The duties, functions and responsibilities of all public health nurses include nursing care and health guidance to persons and families at home, at work, at school and at health centers, as well as collaboration with other professional and citizen groups in planning and activating the community health program and the educational program for nurses and their coworkers.[67] In a few states, such as Iowa and South Dakota, the Public Health Laws and Regulations may be interpreted as giving the nurse a little more leeway in what she can do. For example, she may conduct the physical examinations of children in the public schools. Inasmuch as at law, government agencies may not be liable for damages of employees in the absence of a statutory provision for the same, and since a government cannot be sued without the express consent of the government, the employee himself may be the only one from whom a recovery in damages for negligent or wrongful acts may be obtained.

Again, the public health staff nurse is reminded of the necessity and value of keeping adequate and accurate records. For example, in one case, a visiting nurse's records were used as evidence in an action.[68]

The comparatively recent case of *Denver v. Pollard*[69] has significance for all occupational and public health nurses. In that case, a public health nurse employed by the City and County of Denver came in close physical contact with individuals infected with beta streptococcus. When she became infected, suffered from acute rheumatic fever and was forced to leave her work in January 1963, she brought a suit before the Industrial Commission. Her employers were ordered to pay her weekly compensation for the period of her disability.

In another case, in which a public health nurse was assaulted and sustained a dislocated shoulder, facial cuts and bruises inflicted by a person residing in the home of a patient being visited, he was tried and convicted of assault with intent to commit rape.[70]

Some years ago, a local welfare department nurse's license was revoked for acts derogatory to the morals and standing of the profession of nursing.[71] This particular nurse visited patients without the knowledge and consent of their doctors and without the patients' request. She also told some of them that their diagnoses were incorrect and gave her own. In addition, there was evidence that she had used unwarranted and unprofessional language in criticizing patients and doctors.

Regan reports that a U.S. public health nurse was held liable when serious nerve injury resulted from her carelessly administered infusion while assisting in a mass inoculation program following a devastating flood in a midwestern community.[72]

The school nurse who works alone much of the time and does not have a physician nearby for ready consultation must still use prudence and report the observations she makes in the course of discharging her duty to the physician. Regan[73] reports that when a school nurse informed a girl's parents and the school principal of what appeared to be a venereal disease, and a later medical examination reported a negative finding, she was sued for defamation of character.

Several recent decisions may affect the work of the public health nurse. The United States Court of Appeals decided that a manufacturer of Sabin polio vaccine could be held liable for damages to an adult who contracted paralytic poliomyelitis apparently as a result of receiving Sabin Type III vaccine in a mass immunization program.[74] It held that the drug company had a duty to warn people, either itself or through purchasers, of the dangers involved in taking the vaccine. How this decision will affect mass immunization programs is yet not certain. The regional medical programs will likely benefit from another decision, in which the court required an anesthesiologist practicing in a smaller city to meet the general standard of care applicable to all specialists in his field regardless of where they were located.[75] Furthermore, the court stated that it would apply this rule to general practitioners.

The crux of the public health or visiting nurses' problems lies in good judgment and adequate written nursing policies which define the limits of services. For example, by the Englewood Visiting Nurse Service policies:

> The nurse is forbidden to catheterize male patients, give allergic preparations, bismuth injections, codified drugs, curare, gold compounds, nitrogen mustard.[76]

In the same way, the Visiting Nurse Service of New York allows only two visits to a patient without medical supervision.[77] Such matters as verbal orders, reporting of a patient's condition, giving of injections, procedure in an anaphylactic reaction, special instructions in regard to certain medicines and procedures and so forth are covered in the Englewood model policy.

When students are working under the supervision of nurses in the agency, then under the master-servant doctrine (*respondeat su-*

perior) the agency can be held liable if they negligently injure some patient. When a college or university sends its own instructor with nursing students who care for patients in the agency, and she is in control of the students, it is likely that the instructor and college or university would be liable if the student nurse negligently injures a patient. On the other hand, if the agency is, to some appreciable extent, jointly in control of the nursing students, then it could also be held liable.

Recording telephone orders on a form, dating them and sending them to the physician for written confirmation is probably a method that helps considerably to secure written orders. The necessity for securing written consents for treatment of minors or for photographs of patients is the same in public health as in the hospital; they must be obtained. The Visiting Nurse Service of New York extended its liability insurance to cover the activities of volunteers who took patients out-of-doors and also invited their legal counsel representatives from the State Board of Examiners of Nurses to meet with representatives of the administrative staff and director of the home aide program to make certain the home aide program was on a sound legal basis.

Public health nurses and others who use agency or hospital automobiles will find the case of *Sadler v. Draper*[78] instructive. An action was brought for damages for personal injuries sustained from being struck by a Ford automobile owned by Sadler in charge of his employee Foxhall and driven by Crenshaw. The plaintiff charged that the dealer via his employee acting in the scope of his employment negligently entrusted the automobile to another driver knowing that the driver was unfit, reckless and a habitual drunkard, and that the negligence of the dealer through his employee was the cause of the injuries sued for. The award of $85,000 for multiple fractures of pelvic bones, hip joints, a punctured bladder and multiple compound fractures of both legs was upheld. Various agency policies limiting the use of automobiles to certain drivers, and in some instances rather strictly limiting the passengers who may be transported in such agency cars, are related to the agency's liability and liability insurance coverage and should be adhered to.

Teaching and Administrative Nurses

The writer has found no cases involving nurses as teachers and educational administrators, but believes that such nurses would be considered employees of the institution engaging their services. The personal liability of employees as well as their ability to render the employer liable for negligent and wrongful acts in the scope of their employment has been discussed. As employees, teachers and educational administrators have the same rights as other employees on contract and under the Social Security and compensation laws.

Though such persons may have more education, training and experience in their profession than the average nurse, the employer's right to control their actual performance of the details of their work is the chief basis for believing that such nurses are employees.

Industrial Nurses

The industrial nurse who is engaged by a company or private corporation to render nursing services to its employees is usually regarded as an employee either on the basis of the master-servant rule or on the theory that the corporation has the authority to control the details of the performance of the service. For example, when a patient sued a corporation in an action for damage caused by the negligent acts of a physician, the court said that when the acts were solely for the benefit of the employer's business the master may be liable for the negligent acts of a physician acting in his interest.[79] If the acts complained of had been those of a nurse rather than a physician, it would seem that the same result would be obtained. However, in New York it would seem otherwise; that is, that an industrial nurse would be regarded as an independent contractor in matters relating to the patient's care, and hence the corporation would not be liable for damages to a patient suffering injuries due to a nurse's negligence. In such a case the industrial nurse may be the corporation's agent, but an agent who is an independent contractor does not make a principal liable for his actions in carrying out the details of a contract, since control over such details remains with the agent.[80]

In the case of industrial nurses, the problem of "standing orders" arises. Here, the nurse must be careful to limit her work to the practice of nursing. The industrial nurse must realize that no matter who writes the standing orders, he cannot give the nurse the right or license to practice medicine.[81]

An employee brought a lawsuit for damages against a company and an industrial nurse for malpractice arising out of her treatment of a puncture wound he sustained in the forehead. At the time of the accident, he went to the dispensary, and she swabbed and bandaged the wound but did not probe it for possible foreign matter. Eventually, the wound healed, but a small red area remained, and it began to spread and become puffy. After 10 months' treatment, he requested the nurse to send him to the doctor. A laboratory examination showed a malignant growth which was removed by surgery. The nurse and her employer were both held liable in damages. The court said:

> Good nursing practice required the nurse to examine the wound for foreign bodies, and if splinters were too deeply embedded, to send the patient to a doctor. . . . The nurse should have realized that a wound which would not heal was one of the seven danger signs of cancer.[82]

Office Nurses

The office nurse engaged by a physician, surgeon or dentist is usually regarded as an employee. The fact that the physician supplies the place of work and the equipment and materials necessary, pays her salary and directs her in the performance of her nursing services is usually such control as is considered to establish an employer-employee relationship. In this situation, the employer as well as the nurse employee may be liable for injury or wrong committed by the nurse. For example, when a patient at the suggestion of a doctor submitted to diathermic treatment by the physician's employee, and that employee, after adjusting the electrodes on the patient's body, left the room, and after the lapse of some time returned and turned off the electricity, having forgotten about the patient, so that the patient was burned, the physician was liable to the patient in damages for injuries caused by the negligence of the employee.[83] However, in another case, in which the nurse was under the direction and control of a surgeon during an operation, and he ordered a one per cent procaine solution, and a solution of formaldehyde was negligently prepared in its place and given to him for use, the court held that the surgeon was entitled to rely on the care and skill of trained nurses and similar persons and was not liable for such negligence.[84] The same result, it would seem, would hold in the case of an office nurse whom the employer selected with due care and in the absence of any information putting him on notice as to her lack of competence. When a woman who had brought her child to a physician's office was requested by the office nurse to assist in holding another child on an x-ray table during examination, and in so doing was injured by burns and a fall, she recovered damages from the physician for the harm caused by the nurse's negligence.[85] In a case in which a doctor's office assistant, who was a high school graduate and who had worked previously as an aide in a hospital for two years, treated a patient involved in an accident in a sheet metal factory on 12 out of 17 visits by soaking, bathing and rebandaging a badly injured hand, and the patient sustained permanent damage, the court held that the care of the physician and his assistant was not comparable with that ordinarily given in the community.[86]

In an action against a physician and his office nurse, an award of $25,000 for the death of a 22-month-old boy was held not excessive when he died apparently from aspirating vomitus when left unattended on his back by the nurse.[87] Earlier in the morning, the child had been treated by the physician, and was brought back to the office by his mother, who thought he was much worse. She told the nurse that she believed the child had a convulsion. When the office nurse called the doctor, she told him the child seemed to be in about the same condition as earlier in the day, so the doctor had his lunch before returning to the office. Then the office nurse went to lunch, leaving the receptionist in charge. Some minutes later, the child vomited while lying on his back on the treatment table, and died within a few minutes. A policeman uncle who happened to come in was unsuccessful in reviving him with artificial respiration. Had the nurse been present when the child vomited, there were a number of things she could have done, such as turn him on his side, extract the vomitus and, in an emergency, give a stimulant. An outline of the functions and duties of an office nurse as set forth by the American Nurses' Association shows that her duties include carrying out doctor's orders, nursing procedures, charting and recording, and health guidance and supervision and direction of ancillary workers.[88]

Practical Nurses

Next, we may consider further the status of a practical nurse. As discussed in Chapter II, the practical nurse is one prepared to share in the care of the sick, in rehabilitation, and in prevention of illness, always under the care of a licensed physician and/of a registered professional nurse. The practical nurse, like any other nurse, is responsible for her own wrongful and negligent acts. For example, if a practical nurse applied a hot water bottle to a patient and the patient was burned, the practical nurse would be liable; her power of observation and attention to detail, even without elaborate training, would prevent such results. She may not exceed her authority in the practice of nursing, and she is liable for unauthorized practice of medicine.[89] The provisions of the licensure act and the extent of her education and training in an approved school are factors governing her practice of nursing.

Though the practical nurse may be employed and give nursing care in private homes, institutions and health agencies to a variety of chronically ill, aged or convalescent patients, she is reminded that she works only under direct orders of a licensed physician or under the supervision of a registered professional nurse. For her own protection, as well as that of her patient, the practical nurse should be careful to observe such limitation in practice. The practical nurse, as well as the professional nurse, must realize that no one can give her the right to do more than she is authorized by law to do.

In particular, she should realize that the scarcity of available professional registered nurses does not permit her or technicians or aides to carry out functions which are recognized as within the exclusive area of registered professional nursing.[90] The tendency of some hospitals, nursing homes and other institutions to ask the practical nurse and others to carry out duties beyond the scope of their educational preparation, experience and licensure is to be deplored. In event of a lawsuit, the practical nurse who, along with all others, is responsible for her own actions, will find herself in difficulties if she has assumed the responsibilities of a registered professional nurse, since one who assumes such a role is held to the standard of performance of the registered professional nurse.[91] In some institutions, this problem is particularly acute on the evening and night tours of duty.

Following a prostatectomy, the patient's doctor telephoned the hospital and gave an order for Levophed to the practical nurse, who was the only one on duty on that unit at the time. He neglected to warn her about the drug or to state that only a resident physician should administer the drug. When the patient sustained permanent arm damage as a result of an improper transfusion or failure to keep the needle in place, a sizable award against the hospital was upheld. On the grounds that he was entitled to rely on the competency of the hospital staff in carrying out his order, the doctor was ruled not liable.[92] The practical nurse, like any other employee, renders her employer as well as herself liable for her negligent acts in the course of her employment.

The practical nurse may sue or be sued for breach of a contract for personal services. The same rules for the negotiation and performance of contracts apply to her as to others. For example, if a patient fails to pay her wages or dismisses her in breach of contract, the practical nurse has a cause of action. In an emergency, a practical nurse, like any other person, may give medical care. But again, the practical nurse is reminded that whether there is an emergency in fact depends on all the circumstances.

Aides, Orderlies and Attendants

Aides, orderlies and attendants, as is true of everyone, are responsible at law for their own actions, including negligence. In addition, when a person is injured by an aide, orderly or attendant as a result of negligence in the course of the employee's work, the employer is responsible to the injured person. In a case in which a patient who had almost recovered from a sciatic nerve injury was being taken to the physical therapy department by a nurse's aide who lost control of the stretcher on a ramp, so that it rolled around, overturned and dumped the patient on the floor, the patient recovered for his injuries.[93]

When a patient who had undergone eye surgery was being moved from one hospital building to another, and the stretcher slipped while being lifted by an ambulance attendant and a hospital attendant whose help he had recruited, and the patient's eye was injured as a result, he could not recover damages on the basis of negligence on the grounds that the city ordinance required the ambulance to have two attendants. The court held that the ordinance was concerned only with the cleanliness of drivers and their ability to give first aid, hence both the hospital and ambulance company were found not liable for damages.[94]

When a paying patient, who was blind and partially paralyzed, was taken in a wheelchair by an orderly to a bathroom and, while being prepared for a bath, fell against a steam radiator and sustained third degree burns, allegedly because the orderly went for help instead of moving the patient immediately, the patient was allowed to sue the voluntary hospital for negligence.[95] The patient charged that the charitable hospital was negligent in employing and retaining the services of the orderly, who was incompetent for the work and who had been released from the penitentiary only a few weeks prior, after serving a sentence of several years for conviction of a felony.

A patient signaled for a nurse and asked the nurse's aide who came if she could go to the bathroom. The aide said she could go and handed the patient her slippers and housecoat. The unattended patient was seriously injured in a fall shortly thereafter, and was allowed to recover damages.[96] The stroke patient who suffered a broken leg while being turned by a nurse's aide in a hospital bed recovered substantial damages.[97] When a patient sued for injuries incurred while being catheterized by an orderly in the hospital, the state supreme court reversed a judgment for the defendant hospital and ordered a new trial, in which three urologists testified that the injury was due to the failure of the orderly to use the catheter properly.[98]

In a case in which warm compresses properly applied aggravated a pre-existing cellulitis and infection which had symptoms similar to a second degree burn, the nurse's aide and her employer were cleared in a lawsuit claiming damages for negligence resulting in burns.[99]

The small pamphlet, *A Guide for Assigning Responsibilities,*[100] prepared by the South Dakota Board of Nursing to assist the staff in hospitals, nursing homes, doctors' offices and other health agencies who assign responsibilities to nursing personnel, is an example of the clarification many nurses need on this topic. While the definitions, functions and interpretations given are applicable to that state, it shows what a State Board of Nursing cooperating with a State Nurses' Association, State League for Nursing and Licensed Practical Nurse Association did to help solve this problem.

Student Nurses

In cases arising from the negligent acts of student nurses in a hospital situation, the student nurse has generally been considered an employee and the hospital-employer liable under the master-servant rules. It is important for the student nurse, as is true of other persons, to remember that she is personally liable for her own wrongs and negligent acts. The fact that she is a student and may be a "minor" in reard to age does not exempt her from liability or responsibility for her actions. If the student nurse enjoys employee status, she may make others liable, too, for her negligent acts. In cases which come to trial, the facts relating to the student nurse's admission, her experience record, and her efficiency ratings may be presented in detail for consideration as to whether she acted like an ordinary, reasonable, prudent student nurse under the circumstances.[101]

In a case in which two student nurses during an influenza epidemic received a head nurse's permission to give nursing care to a child during off-duty hours, and the child received burns from a lighted alcohol inhalator, the court held that the student nurses were directly acting within the scope of their employment and the hospital was liable for actual damages.[102] In another case, a charitable hospital was held liable to a private duty nurse for damages for injuries resulting from the negligent act of a student nurse in the regular employment of the hospital.[103] In other cases, whether a patient may recover from a hospital for injuries caused by negligent acts of student nurses depends on the status of the employer as one who operates a governmental, charitable or private institution. Accordingly, when a patient was burned by an excessively hot hypodermoclysis through the negligence of a student nurse, it was held that the only obligation a charitable institution owes the public is to select with due care the persons who act as nurses.[104] In a city hospital in which a paying patient suffered serious personal injuries as a result of the negligence of a student nurse employed by the hospital, the city was held not liable to the patient since conducting the hospital was an exercise of its governmental power.[105]

The parents of a newborn baby recovered damages for her wrongful death when a heating lamp with an unguarded bulb was placed by a student nurse within three inches of the bed clothing. Somewhat later she discovered the baby's bassinet enveloped in flames.[106] When a student nurse disregarded a warning on an ampule that stated that the drug was for intravenous use only, and she injected the medicine into an infant's buttock, and as a result a crippling injury occurred in the corresponding leg, the parents sued the physicians and settled out of court for $10,000 damages.[107] A patient received a judgment against a hospital and its student nurse when he lost his leg due to the carelessness of the student nurse in using an electric pad.[108] The patient was heavily sedated and during the night the electric pad burned the leg so severely it had to be amputated.

When nursing students in the course of their clinical experience in hospitals or other agencies perform duties that are within the scope of professional nursing, these acts must be performed with the same degree of competence as if done by a registered professional nurse. In other words, the patient must not be subjected to a lower standard of nursing care because he has nursing students caring for him. When a nursing student is negligent in the performance of her duties, the patient may bring a lawsuit for damages.

It is pertinent to point out that an instructor is responsible for her assignments and for reasonable and prudent supervision of nursing students. Accordingly, if she were to assign a nursing student to perform duties for which she had not been trained, or were to neglect or omit supervising her performance to ascertain that she was competent at a professional level, the instructor could be held liable. The inherent responsibility of the nurse who supervises others — whether it is nursing students, registered professional nurses, practical nurses, aides, orderlies, or attendants — is to determine which of the patient's needs can be safely entrusted to a particular person and whether or not the person to whom the duty is delegated or assigned is competent only if personally supervised. An integral part of a clinical instructor's duty is to supervise the fitness and competency of nursing students who give nursing care to patients, and any negligence in failing to supervise in accordance with the standard of a reasonable and prudent clinical instructor is the basis of liability.[109]

When a first-year student in a hospital in which first-year students were permitted to give injections under supervision, gave one to a patient hospitalized with Buerger's disease, and injured his right sciatic nerve, the patient recovered a substantial judgment because the defendant hospital had not provided adequate supervision.[110]

The nursing student should bear in mind that he or she is responsible for his or her own actions and is liable for his or her own negligence.[111] The fact that some nursing students are under 21 years of age does not change or lessen their potential liability. As has been pointed out in the preceding discussion, the nursing student will be required to adhere to the same standard of care as the ordinary, reasonable and prudent professional nurse. Consequently, if a nursing student knows that he is inadequately prepared for a particular assignment or duty or needs additional supervision, he should inform the person responsible for his assignment and supervision of the matter.

In past years, the nursing student in a diploma program in a hospital school of nursing was considered an employee of the hospital when she was doing nursing in the institution, under its direction and for its benefit.[112] In a recent case, the nursing student was compared to an apprentice, and the court held that the relationship of employer and employee existed.[113] When such a nursing student was assigned by her school to an affiliated hospital for special training, she was still considered to be an employee who had both a general and a special employer.[114] In the case of a nursing student under the United States Cadet Nurse Corps nurse training program at a university who contracted a disease that disabled her, compensation from the university as the employer was awarded. The university paid her a monthly stipend and retained control over students, and the affiliating hospitals supplied room, board, laundry and practical training.[115] When in the course of her duties, a third-year student nurse was putting a box of vials containing acid back in the closet, and she sustained acid burns on her legs when it broke, she was held to be an employee of the hospital and her only remedy was under the Workmen's Compensation Law.[116]

However, the nursing student may not be an employee. Today the nursing students in associate degree and collegiate programs typically receive no stipend from the college. The nursing students provide their own room, board and laundry and usually pay some tuition fees. When the nursing students are in the hospital practice area, the faculty of the college teaches them and the hospital simply provides for clinical experience without giving any compensation to the student or making any service demands. In such instances, the nursing student would not seem to be an employee of the hospital, but might be held to be an employee of the college. A patient who suffered injuries as a result of manipulation by a student of osteopathy recovered damages from the college, and the court said that a student in a clinical situation must be given reasonable guidance and supervision.[117]

Not only may the student nurse incur personal liability and make others also liable by reason of her acts, but she also has rights. Thus, a student nurse who contracted tuberculosis while she was in contact with tubercular patients in the course of her hospital duties was entitled to compensation.[118] As previously pointed out, the student nurse was expressly exempted by law from the Social Security program.

In view of the recent trend in some collegiate institutions for student nurses to pay substantial sums for their education and to render more limited amounts of nursing care in hospitals, and that for "educational purposes" rather than the rendering of service in exchange for maintenance and training, future cases involving student nurses might not consider them employees of the hospital when caring for patients.

At this point, it should be apparent to the nurse that existing laws relating to her profession seek to protect the nurses as well as the general public. The nurse should have no fear in practicing her profession so far as legal matters are concerned. Rather, she should become grounded in the various legalities as they apply to her work and daily living, so that she approaches her tasks with complete confidence.

MALPRACTICE INSURANCE

A good feature for nurses to look into is the matter of insurance. Nurses' malpractice or professional liability insurance pays the damages (to the extent of the face value of the policy) if any are awarded by the court, and it also provides expert legal counsel to defend a claim and pays the cost of such defense. Such policies may be secured in amounts ranging from $5000/$15,000 upward for a relatively small insurance premium. A $5000/$15,000 policy means that the insurance company will pay up to $5000 in damages to any one person who is injured as a result of the nurse's real or alleged malpractice; and it will pay up to $15,000 in damages in any one year on all claims involving the insured nurse. It is the view of many authorities that all registered nurses should carry malpractice insurance to cover the cost of expert legal counsel and to pay possible claims for damages. At times, it has been necessary for a nurse to prove that she was not negligent, and this litigation can be costly.

When the representatives of the insurance carrier declined to accept a pre-trial offer to settle out of court for $45,000 in a malpractice suit which came to trial and resulted in a $120,000 judgment, a physician whose policy covered him only up to $70,000 succeeded in making his insurance carrier pay $50,000 more than his policy coverage.[119]

An employee cannot always rely on his employer's insurance. Sometimes a nurse may feel more secure than the facts warrant when she thinks that her employer's malpractice insurance will cover the personal liability of the employed nurse. This is seldom the case, according to the findings of a recent article.[120] The nurse desiring protection should take out her own malpractice insurance. The American Nurses' Association sponsors a group plan which is available to any member on an individual basis. Some of the states have group plans, such as the California State Nurses' Association.

The recent changing patterns of a nurse's activities contribute to her increased exposure to lawsuits. A number of years ago, the court held that it was a matter of common knowledge that the welfare of the patient was as much the responsibility of the nurse as of the physician.[121] Today, when nurses are asked to and do carry out a great variety of procedures, give many new drugs and are responsible for the supervision or teaching of assorted personnel and patients, there are increased legal responsibilities. Then, too, this is an age of specialists; for example, nurses give care in Coronary Care Units and in Intensive Care Units where patients may receive organ transplants, undergo renal dialysis, receive hyperbaric care or receive treatment for severe neurologic or other problems. The nurse who is thus engaged as a specialist is expected to possess the qualifications of a person ordinarily practicing in that speciality. Although in some states, the nurses' association, the hospital association and the medical association have worked together constructively to delineate what the professional nurse may do by way of nursing care in critical patient care situations, other states have taken no action to clarify the grey area between nursing and medical practice.

JOINT POLICY STATEMENTS

The following joint statement is an example of constructive effort to clarify for legal purposes a new procedure expected of nurses:

Joint Policy Statement Concerning the Role of Professional Registered Nurses Practicing in New Hampshire in Administering Closed Chest Cardio-Pulmonary Resuscitation.

NEW HAMPSHIRE HOSPITAL ASSOCIATION
NEW HAMPSHIRE MEDICAL SOCIETY
NEW HAMPSHIRE NURSES' ASSOCIATION

With the objective of protecting the patient, the doctor, the nurse, and the employer, the New Hampshire Nurses' Association, the New Hampshire Medical Association and the New Hampshire Hospital Association acknowledge their acceptance of the right of Registered Nurses to carry out the procedures of "Closed Chest Cardio-Pulmonary Resuscitation" if all of the following conditions exist:

1. The nurse has had special competent instruction in carrying out the procedure of "Closed Chest Cardio-Pulmonary Resuscitation," and
2. The nurse has had competent teaching in the technique including the recognition, understanding and interpretation of the symptoms of cardiac arrest, and
3. A physician is not immediately available to initiate the procedure, and
4. The physician is notified immediately, and
5. The physician upon his arrival assumes the responsibility for the procedure.

Where the procedure is to be performed in a hospital or any organized agency, it is to be performed within the framework of:

A. Policies established for the regulation of "Closed Chest Cardio-Pulmonary Resuscitation" and the preparation of the nurse. It is recommended that the policies be established by a committee composed of representatives of the Medical staff, the Nursing staff and the agency administration. The policies to be written and made available to the total medical and nursing staffs.
B. The individual nurse must exercise her professional judgment in determining her qualification and competency to perform this procedure. *Qualifications* and *competency* as herein used implies knowledge of cause and effect in performing this procedure.
C. It is important for each nurse to note that this policy statement will not provide immunity if the practitioner is negligent. The nurse should realize and be aware that any policy statement made by the professional organization or by the employing agency does not relieve him/her of responsibility for his/her acts.

It is recognized that it is the prerogative of the hospital or agency to:

1. Determine if this is a nursing function in their institution.
2. Decide if the nurse may perform the procedure.

3. Determine the method of implementing instruction.
4. Establish in-service teaching of the procedure.
5. Determine the procedural guidelines for "Closed Chest Cardio-Pulmonary Resuscitation."

Note: Nurse means Registered Nurses only.

Approved and signed
NEW HAMPSHIRE NURSES' ASSOCIATION
NEW HAMPSHIRE HOSPITAL ASSOCIATION
NEW HAMPSHIRE MEDICAL SOCIETY
February 1, 1967

A further Joint Statement on the Role of the Registered Nurse in Acute Cardiac Care, as agreed upon by the California Medical Association, California Hospital Association and California Nurses' Association, states:

We recognize the propriety of registered nurses to use monitoring, defibrillation, and resuscitative equipment, and to institute immediate life-saving corrective measures, if a licensed physician is not immediately available to do so and the following conditions exist:

1. The registered nurse has had special competent instruction in the techniques.
2. The registered nurse performs the authorized procedures upon:
   a. the direct order of a licensed doctor of medicine, or
   b. pursuant to standing procedures established as set forth in item 4 following.
3. Where a hospital has determined that a registered nurse may perform the techniques, then the techniques to be performed within the framework of designated preparation and practice of the nurse shall be established for the hospital by a committee composed of representatives from the medical staff, the department of nursing, and the administration. Thus the framework of preparation and practice shall be reproduced in writing and made available to the total medical and nursing staffs.
4. Such criteria shall make provision that in case of a cardiac emergency, a licensed physician and other designated categories of personnel are to be immediately summoned to assist the registered nurse who is carrying out the physician's orders or is carrying out standing procedures established by the medical staff of the hospital, and contained in the adopted criteria.
5. It is the jurisdiction of that Committee in a hospital or organized agency to:
   a. decide if the nurses in the hospital or agency may perform the technique,
   b. determine the special method of teaching to be required,
   c. establish inservice teaching of the technique for any nurses who may not have had adequate previous instruction,
   d. delineate the solutions which may be given safely with blood, and delineate the types of fluids or medications

that nurses may administer intravenously, including medications to be put into fluid or any part of the equipment being used in the administration of the IV fluids,

e. determine whether physicians' orders should be written or oral (such determination to be consistent with the hospital or agency's rules regarding written confirmation of oral orders).[122]

While there have been few charges against nurses who have expanded their area of practice and few charges against physicians who have delegated these new functions to nurses, it does not lessen the desirability of a nurse's being protected against a lawsuit. Each nurse should have her own liability or malpractice insurance.

In special units, such as a C.C.U. or an I.C.U., there should be written policies to be followed in the event that cardiac standstill or some other problem occurs. These policies which affect the practice of nursing should be written by a committee which includes registered professional nurses. Nursing practice should be controlled by nurses, but if this is to be achieved nurses must act collectively on the practice issue, and as Jacox has pointed out, they may get more resistance from hospital administrators on this point than on economic issues.[123] Nurses should review carefully the nursing practice act of the state in which they work and look to their professional organization to take leadership in securing joint statements of policy like those cited. As Anderson has stated:

> The only group permitted by law to interpret what constitutes the legal practice of nursing is the State Board of Nursing, composed of state appointed government officials acting to protect the public.[124]

The Code for Professional Nurses has two statements that bear on such work:

> The nurse assumes responsibility for individual professional actions and judgments, both in dependent and independent nursing functions, and knows and upholds the laws which affect the practice of nursing.
> The fundamental responsibility of the nurse is to conserve life, to alleviate suffering, and to promote health.

Whether student nurses should be allowed to render any nursing service in an Intensive Care Unit is questioned by many legal authorities. If they give any service, they should be closely supervised.

It is important that nurses' notes should be taken frequently and should describe in detail what takes place. One sample of excellent and pertinent charting covering an emergency situation is the flow chart given by Duke.[125]

As a precaution in matters of evidence, the special preparation and advanced education of nurses working in a special unit should be on record in their personnel file. Whenever a nurse takes additional training or courses, it is her responsibility to keep her record up-to-date.

In addition, it is helpful for nurses to maintain records showing that equipment used in the special units is routinely checked as being in good working order. The mechanical failure of any equipment is possible, and nurses must be alert for such contingencies and must be prepared to take appropriate action.

REFERENCES

1. Ranelli v. Society of New York Hospital, 56 N.Y.S. 2d 481, Aff'm., 295 N.Y. 850, 67 N.E. 2d 257 (App. Div. 2d Dept. 1946). See also Necolayff v. Genesee Hospital, 296 N.Y. 936, 73 N.E. 2d 117 (Sup. Ct., App. T. 1947)
2. Pierson v. Charles S. Wilson Memorial Hospital, 273 App. Div. 348, 78 N.Y.S. 146 (1948)
3. Fowler v. State, 78 N.Y.S. 2d 860 (Ct. Cl. 1948)
4. 2 Restatement, Torts, § 314
5. Malloy v. Fong, 37 Cal. 2d 356, 220 P 2d 48, 233 P 2d 241 (1951)
5a. Cf. Question for Good Samaritan; Is This Emergency Really Real? Ohio Nurses Rev., 41:13-14, Jan., 1966
6. Creighton, Helen: Legal Responsibilities of the R.N. in the Emergency Room. Mississippi RN, 30:35-40, Oct., 1968. Lamberten, Eleanor C.: Education for Nursing Leadership. Philadelphia, J. B. Lippincott Co., 1958, pp. 165-6
7. Social Security Administration. Document HIM-1. p. 35, 1966
8. Letourneau, Charles U.: Legal Aspects of the Hospital Emergency Room. Hospital Management, 103:55-60, Mar., 1967; 103:39-41, Apr., 1967
9. Wilmington General Hospital v. Manlove, 54 Del. 15, 174 A 2d 135 (1961)
10. O'Neill v. Montefiore Hospital, et al., 11 A.D. 2d 231, 202 N.Y.S. 2d 436 (1960)
11. Ruvio v. North Broward Hospital District, 186 So. 2d 45 (1966)
12. American College of Surgeons: Standards for the Emergency Department. Approved by the Board of Regents, Feb. 23-24, 1963
13. Creighton, Helen: Legal Responsibilities of the R.N. in the Emergency Room. Mississippi RN, 30:35-40, Oct., 1968
14. American Nurses' Association: Statement of Functions. Am. J. Nursing, 54:868-71, 994-6, 1130, 1954
15. People ex rel. Burke v. Steinberg, 73 N.Y.S. 2d 475 (Mag. Ct. N.Y.C. 1947)
16. Thomson v. Virginia Mason Hospital, 152 Wash. 297, 277 Pac. 691 (1929)
17. Education Law, N.Y. Consolidated Laws Service (Issue 2, 1955) Tit. 8, Art. 131, § 6512, ¶ 21, 22, 1(j)
18. Byrd v. Marion General Hospital, 202 N.C. 337, 162 N.E. 738 (1932)
19. Parrish v. Clark, 107 Fla. 598, 145 So. 848 (1933). See also Wood v. Miller, 158 Ore. 444, 76 P 2d 963 (1938)
20. Morrison v. Henke, 165 Wis. 166, 160 N.W. 173 (1916)
21. Hayt, Emanuel, et al.: Law of Hospital and Nurse. New York, Hospital Textbook Co., 1958, p. 320
22. Forestel v. United States, 261 F. Supp. 269 (1966)
23. Cf. Regan, William A.: Telephone Orders and Legal Risks. Regan Report on Nursing Law, 8(1)1, June, 1967; Nursing Judgment vs. Medical Judgment. Regan Report on Nursing Law, 9(4)1, Sept., 1968; Nurses, Diagnosis and the Law. Regan Report on Nursing Law, 8(5) 1, Oct. 1967
24. People of the State of California v. King, 72 Cal. Rptr. 478 (Cal., 1968)
25. Stead, Eugene A.: Training and Use of Paramedical Personnel. New Eng. J. Med., 277:800 ff. Oct. 12, 1967. Darley, Ward, and Somers, Anne R.: Increasing Personnel. New. Eng. J. Med., 276:1414-23, June, 1967. Darley, Ward, and Somers, Anne R.: New Training for New Needs. New Eng. J. Med., 276:1471-8, June 29, 1967. Solomon, Mardoqueo I.: Medical Assistants or Quasi-Physicians. New Eng. J. Med., 277:1373, Dec. 21, 1967. Estes, E. Harvey: Advantages and Limitations of Medical Assistants. J. Am. Geriatr. Soc., 16:1083-7, Oct., 1968. Creating New

Help for Busy MD's. *Med. World News,* 9:16-7, July 12, 1968. Parental Acceptance of Delegated Pediatric Services. *Pediatrics,* 41:1003-4, May, 1968

26. Knisely, William H.: Can Nurses Stand for Doctors? *Med. World News,* 8:82-3; Nov. 27, 1967
27. Vannah v. Hart Private Hospital, 228 Mass. 132, 117 N.E. 328 (1917) See also Gray, Albert W.: Protecting Patients' Property. *Mod. Hosp.,* 78:58 (Feb., 1952)
28. Yohalem v. Yasuma, 165 Misc. 435, 300 N.Y.S. 929 (N.Y. City Ct., 1937)
29. 2 Rev. Stat. Maine c. 69, § 7 (1954); Snelson v. Culton, 141 Me. 242, 42 A. 2d 505 (1945)
30. Burrell, Howard: Legal Hazards of Inadequate Hospital Records. *Mod. Hosp.,* 66:70-2 (March, 1946)
31. Greyhound Corp. v. Superior Court of State of California in and for the County of Merced 15 Cal. Rptr. 90; 364 P 2d 266 (1961)
32. Spoar v. Fudjack, 24 A.D. 2d 731, 263 N.Y.S. 2d 340 (1965)
33. Engle v. Clarke, 346 S.W. 13 (Ct. of Appeals of Ky., 1961)
34. Soto v. State, 55 Misc. 2d 1035, 286 N.Y.S. 993 (1968)
35. *Op. cit. supra,* note 31
36. Gabriel, A.: Medico-Legal Cases on Nurses' Charting. *St. Tomas Nurs. J.,* 5: 273-4, Dec., 1966
37. Fullerton, Donald T., May, Philip R. A., and White, Ruth: The Unusual Incident Report—a Teaching and Therapeutic Device. *J. Psychia. Nurs.,* 3:258-68, May-June, 1965
38. Hospital of St. Vincent of Paul in City of Norfolk v. Thompson, 116 Va. 101, 81 S.E. 13 (1914)
39. Ballance v. Dunnington. 241 Mich. 383, 217 N.W. 329 (1928)
40. Hebel v. Hinsdale Sanitarium and Hosp., 2 Ill. App. 2d 527, 119 N.E. 2d 506 (1954). The fact situation of this case is similar to, but not identical with, the illustration
41. *Cf.* Dittert v. Fischer, 148 Ore. 366, 36 P 2d 592 (1934)
42. Mayer v. Reyes & Co., 13 CCH Neg. Cases 2d 1475 (La. Ct. of Appeals, 4th Cir.) 1962
43. Puffinberger *et al.* v. Day, Calif. Dist. Ct. of Appeals, No. 6845 (1962)
44. Brockman v. Harpole *et al.,* 444 P 2d 25 (Ore. 1968)
45. 17 C.J.S. 644. *Contracts* § 262: Agreements Exempting from Liability for Negligence
46. Thompson v. Fox, 326 Pa. 209, 192 Atl. 107 (1937)
47. Bowers, Renzo Dee: Legal Hazards for Nurses. *Am. J. Nursing,* 47:523-4 (1947)
48. Wright v. Conway, 34 Wyo. 1, 242 Pac. 1107 (1926); Broz v. Omaha Maternity General Hospital, 96 Neb. 648, 148 N.W. 575 (1914)
49. McCowen v. Sisters of Most Precious Blood of Enid, 208 Okla. 130, 253 P 2d 830 (1953)
50. Minogue v. Rutland Hospital, Inc., 119 Vt. 336, 125 A 2d 796 (1956)
51. Meadows v. Patterson, 21 Tenn. App. 283, 108 S.W. 2d 417 (1937) 19 Tenn. L.R. 368 (1946)
52. Schloendorff v. Society of New York Hospital, 211 N.Y. 125, 105 N.E. 92 (1914)
53. American Nurses' Association: Statement of Functions. *Am. J. Nursing,* 54:868-71, 1954
54. Welsh v. Mercy Hospital *et al.,* 65 Cal. App. 2d 473, 151 P 2d 17 (1944)
55. Regan, William A.: Nurse Shortage Remedies Can Be Risky. *Regan Report on Nursing Law,* 5 (8) 1, Jan., 1965
56. *Op. cit. supra,* note 39 at page 869
57. Brown v. St. Vincent's Hospital, 222 App. Div. 402, 226 N.Y.S. 317 (1928)
58. Canney v. Sisters of Charity of House of Providence, 15 Wash. 2d 325, 130 P 2d 899 (1942)
59. Owen v. Williams, 322 Mass. 356, 77 N.E. 2d 318 (1948)
60. Bowers, Renzo Dee: Legal Status of Private Duty Nurses. *Am. J. Nursing,* 48:624-5 (1948). See also Hughes v. President and Directors of Georgetown College, 33 Fed. Supp. 867, aff'm., 130 F 2d 810 (D.C. Circ., 1942)
61. Emory University v. Shadburn, 47 GA. 643 171 S.E. 192, aff'd 180 S.E. 137 (Ga., 1933). Bugalari, Joseph E.: Courts Put Private Duty Nurses Blunders on Your Doorstep. *Mod. Hosp.* 108:87-9, Jan., 1969
62. Mautino v. Sutter Hospital Ass'n., 296 Pac. 76 (Cal. 1931)

63. Wrenn v. Hillcrest Convalescent Home, 270 N.C. 447, 154 S.E. 2d 483 (1967)
64. 203 A. 2d 511 (Pa., 1966). See also *Nursing Homes,* 15:41, June, 1966
65. Edith A. Anderson Nursing Homes, Inc. v. Bettie Walker, 232 Md. 442, 194 A. 2d 85 (1963)
66. Scofield v. Strain, Mayor *et al.,* State *ex rel.,* Reilly v. Hamrock, Mayor *et al.,* 142 Ohio St. 290, 51 N.E. 2d 1012 (1943)
67. American Nurses' Association: Statement of Functions. *Am. J. Nursing,* 54:870-1 (1954). Public Health Nursing Responsibilities in a Community Health Program. *Pub. Health Nursing,* 41:68-9 (1949)
68. McCarthy v. Maxon, 134 Conn. 170, 55 A 2d 912 (1947)
69. 417 P 2d 231 (Colo., 1966)
70. State v. Hyde, 158 N.W. 2d 134. (Iowa, 1968)
71. Stefanik v. Nursing Educational Committee, 37 A 2d 661 (R.I., 1944)
72. Regan, William A.: Clinical Problem — Public Health Nursing. *Regan Report on Nursing Law,* 5 (11) 4, April, 1965
73. *Idem.*
74. Davis v. Wyeth Laboratories, Inc. and American Home Products Corporation, 399 F. 2d 121 (Ct. of Appeals, 9th Cir., 1968)
75. Brune v. Belinkoff, 235 N.E. 2d 793 (Mass., 1968)
76. Regan, William A.: Legal Problems of the R.N. in the Community. *RN,* 30:72-80, Sept., 1967, p. 75
77. Fillmore, Anne: The Visiting Nurse Service and the Law. *Nurs. Outlook,* 12:28-32, June, 1964, p. 30
78. Sadler v. Draper, 46 Tenn. App. 1, 326 S.W. 2d 148 (1959)
79. Rannard v. Lockheed Aircraft Corp., 26 Cal. 2d 149, 150 P 2d 255; Rev'd., 157 P 2d 1 (1945)
80. *In re* Renouf v. New York Central R.R. Co., 254 N.Y. 349, 173 N.E. 218 (1930)
81. Regan, William A.: Doctor and Patient and the Law. 1956, especially p. 483 ff.
82. Cooper v. National Motor Bearing Co., Inc. 288 P 2d 581 (Cal., 1955)
83. Wemmett v. Mount, 134 Ore. 305, 292 Pac. 93 (1930)
84. Hallinan v. Prindle, 220 Cal. 46, 11 P 2d 426 (modified); 17 Cal. App. 2d 656, 29 P 2d 202 (rev'd); 69 P 2d 1075 (aff'm in part, rev'd in part 1936)
85. Kelly v. Yount, 338 Pa. 190, 12 A 2d 579 (1940)
86. Delany v. Rosenthal, 347 Mass. 143, 81A|2 547, 196 N.E. 2d 878 (1964)
87. Crowe v. Provost. 52 Tn Appeals 397, 374 S.W. 2d 645 (1963)
88. American Nurses' Association: Statement of Functions. *Am. J. Nursing,* 54:995-6 (1954)
89. *Op. cit. supra,* note 15, People *ex rel.* Burke v. Steinberg
90. See Regan, William A.: Surgical Nursing — Current Trends. *Regan Report on Nursing Law,* 6(11) 1, April, 1966; You and the Doctor Shortage. *RN,* 25:52-56, Mar. 1962
91. Barber v. Reiking, 411 P.2d 861 (Wash., 1966). The court said: "In accordance with the public policy of this state, one who undertakes to perform the services of a trained or graduate nurse must have the knowledge and skill possessed by a registered nurse."
92. Baidach v. Linden General Hospital. *Regan Report on Nursing Law,* 2(5)3, Oct., 1961
93. Ray v. Tucson Medical Center, 72 Ariz. 22, 230 P.2d 220 (1951)
94. Boie-Hansen v. Sisters of Charity, 314 P. 2d 189 (Calif., 1957)
95. Adkins v. St. Francis Hospital of Charleston, W.Va., 143 S.E. 2d 154 (W. Va. 1965)
96. Shover v. Iowa Lutheran Hospital. *Regan Report on Nursing Law,* 2 (1) 3, June 1961
97. St. John's Hospital & School of Nursing of Tulsa. v. Chapman, 1967 CCH Neg. 1586 (Okla., 1967). Aff'm.
98. Hyland v. St. Marks Hospital, 1967 CCH Neg. 1442 (Utah, 1967)
99. Clovis v. Hartford Accident, 223 So. 178 (La., 1969)
100. South Dakota Board of Nursing, Mitchell, South Dakota, 1966
101. Miller *et ux.* v. Mohr *et al.,* 198 Wash. 619, 89 P 2d 807, 105 P 2d 32 (1939)
102. Longuy v. La Société Française de Bienfaisance Mutuelle, 52 Cal. App. 370, 198 Pac. 1011 (1921)

103. Hughes v. President and Directors of Georgetown College, 33 Fed. Supp. 867, aff'm. 130 F 2d 810 (D.C. 1942)
104. Foye v. St. Francis Sanitarium and Training School for Nurses, 2 La. App. 305 (1925). St. Paul's Sanitarium v. Williamson, 164 S.W. 36 (Tex. Ct. App. 1914). Bise v. St Luke's Hospital, 181 Wash. 269, 43 P 2d 4 (1935)
105. City of McAllen v. Gartmen *et ux.,* 81 S.W. 2d 147, aff'm., 107 S.W. 2d 879 (Texas Ct. of Appeals, 1937)
106. Cadicamo v. Long Island College Hospital, 308 N.Y. 196, 125 N.Y.S. 2d 632, 127 N.Y.S. 2d 855, 124 N.E. 2d 279 (1954)
107. O'Neil v. Glens Falls Indemnity Co., 35 Am. Law Rep. 452, 310 F. 2d 165 (Nebr., 1962)
108. Piedmont Hospital v. Anderson, 65 Ga. App. 491, 16 S.E. 2d 90 (1941)
109. Lesnik, Milton J., and Anderson, Bernice E.: Nursing Practice and the Law, 2nd ed., Philadelphia, J. B. Lippincott Co., 1955, pp. 270-1
110. Regan, William A.: Your Legal Liability When Supervising. *RN,* 32:44, 68, January, 1969
111. *Cf.* Hershey, Nathan: Student, Instructor, and Liability. *Am. J. Nursing,* 65:122-3, Mar., 1965
112. Hewett v. Woman's Hospital Aid Assn., 73 N.H. 556, 64 A 190 (1906). Bernstein v. Beth Israel Hospital, 236 N.Y. 268, 140 N.E. 694 (1923)
113. Heget v. Christ Hospital, 26 N.J. Misc. 189, 58 A 2d 615 (1948)
114. Cook v. Buffalo General Hospital, 308 N.Y. 480, 127 N.E. 2d 66 (1955)
115. Otto v. State, 40 N.W. 2d 81 (Minn., 1949)
116. Galligan v. St. Vincent's Hospital, 28 App. Div. 2d 592 (1968)
117. Christensen v. Des Moines Still College of Osteopathy, 82 N.W. 2d 741 (Iowa, 1957)
118. McDonough v. Flushing Hospital and Dispensary, 43 N.Y.S. 2d 889 (Sup. Ct., 1943)
119. Price v. Neyland, 320 F. 2d 674 (1963)
120. Barbee, Grace C.: When Is the Nurse Held Liable? *Am. J. Nursing,* 54:1343-6 (1954)
121. Miller v. Mohr, 198 Wash. 619, 89 P 2d 807 (1939)
122. Joint Statement on the Role of the Registered Nurse in Acute Cardiac Care. *CNA Bull.,* 62:5, Mar., 1966. Also, *Calif. Med.,* 104:228, Mar., 1966
123. Jacox, Ada K.: Who Defines and Controls Nursing Practice? *Am. J. Nursing,* 69:977-982, May, 1969
124. Anderson, Bernice E.: Legal Aspects of Nursing Care for Cardiac Patients. *Cardiovascular Nursing,* 5(2) 6, Mar-Apr. 1969
125. Duke, Martin: *JAMA,* 202:143-5, Oct. 9, 1967

General References

Anderson, Bernice E.: Legal Aspects of MCH Nursing. *Virginia Nurse Quarterly,* 36:5-16, Spring, 1968
Barbee, Grace C.: The Nurse, the Nursing Home and the Law. *Am. J. Nursing,* 61:84-86, 1961
Bernzweig, Eli P.: Liability for Malpractice—Its Role in Nursing Education. *J. Nurs. Educ.,* 8:33-41, April, 1969
Functions and Qualifications for School Nurses. *Am. J. Nursing,* 61:93, May, 1961
Hayt, Emanuel, *et al.:* Law of Hospital and Nurse. New York, Hospital Textbook Co., 1958, p. 362 ff.
Hershey, Nathan: Students as Staff Nurses? *Am. J. Nursing,* 67:117, Jan., 1967; Pitfalls in Liability Insurance. *Am. J. Nursing,* 66:2202-3, Sept., 1966; He Can't Take the Responsibility. *Am. J. Nursing,* 66:1053-4, May, 1966; The Office Nurse, *Am. J. Nursing,* 65:108-110, May, 1965
Lesnik, Milton J., and Anderson, Bernice E.: Nursing Practice and the Law, 2d ed., Philadelphia, J. B. Lippincott Co., 1955. See Chap. 8 on Legal Aspects of Negligence and Malpractice, pp. 234-304
Regan, William A.: The Nurse's Role in Emergency Cases. *Regan Report on Nursing Law,* 4 (9) 1, Feb., 1964; You and Experimental Medicine. *RN,* 29:75-79, July, 1966
Wall, Lucille: Legal Aspects of Closed Chest Cardiac Resuscitation. *Indiana Nurse,* 29:25-7, Dec., 1965

Chapter Seven

Negligence and Malpractice

This chapter describes a variety of cases involving negligence or malpractice in the field of nursing so that the nurse may know the basis of some claims against nurses.

DEFINITION OF NEGLIGENCE

Negligence has been defined as the omission to do something which a reasonable person, guided by those ordinary considerations which ordinarily regulate human affairs, would do, or as doing something which a reasonable and prudent person would not do.[1]

DEFINITION OF MALPRACTICE

Malpractice has been defined as any professional misconduct, unreasonable lack of skill or fidelity in professional or judiciary duties, evil practice, or illegal or immoral conduct.[2] Moreover, it would appear desirable that the nurse should understand the meaning of malpractice as it applies to physicians: it means bad, wrong or injudicious treatment resulting in injury, unnecessary suffering, or death to the patient, and proceeding from ignorance, care-

110

lessness, want of proper professional skill, disregard of established rules or principles, neglect or a malicious or criminal intent.[3] Since the nurse is closely associated in her work with the physician, and since malpractice suits are numerous, indeed, if the nurse understands the nature of the problem and the acts of commission or omission that give rise to the suits, she may the better cooperate with physicians and others in minimizing the problem. In a previous chapter, on the matter of the completeness and accuracy of records, it was evident how helpful the nurse could and should be in this matter.

Again, the nurse's attention is called to the fact that generally malpractice suits come from patients who have poor results from treatment. A friendly patient who feels that nurses and doctors have done their best for him is not the one who is likely to sue. Hence, the need for tactful handling of patients who are dissatisfied with their care and progress should be evident to a nurse. Moreover, since the nurse may spend more time than a physician in rendering care to a patient, her handling of a patient and his family may be of great importance. The way she relates to these people may make the difference between a suit and refusal to sue for malpractice against a physician.

One writer, in discussing malpractice and how a physician's office nurse can contribute to the lessening thereof, enumerates seven rules of conduct.[4] The nurse (1) is always polite to patients, regardless of circumstances, (2) does not discuss the patient's ailments with him, (3) does not discuss the respective merits of various forms of therapy, (4) never prescribes, (5) does not discuss other doctors with the patient, (6) keeps a record when the patient does not return as directed, and (7) is alert to hazards. The nurse who observes such rules in her practice, be it in the hospital, the home, a public health agency or elsewhere, will certainly minimize malpractice actions not only against a physician, but also against herself.

Generally, suits based on negligence or malpractice are brought in civil courts to recover damages for the injuries claimed. However, when the negligence or malpractice amounts to wanton and reckless conduct or shows a disregard of human life, the law regards it as criminal and the action is handled in criminal courts. Discussion and illustration of the latter classification are reserved for the next chapter.

Malpractice claims give rise to such questions as whether or not the nurse is solely responsible for the alleged act, omission or other wrongs, and how the physician and hospital are implicated, if at all. A point for the nurse to remember is that in states in which the governmental or voluntary charitable institution is exempt from liability, the injured patient has only the nurse, doctor or other individual from whom he may seek to recover damages for his alleged negligently caused injury.

LIABILITY FOR NEGLIGENCE

Everyone has a duty to behave as a reasonably prudent person would act in the particular circumstances. This means that an individual must handle himself and his property so as to avoid injury to the person or property of others. In a civil action for damages based on negligence, the person sued must have done or failed to do some act which he was under a duty to do and there must be an injury to the person bringing suit which can be traced directly to the breach of this duty. For example, in New York a parent sued a physician and a hospital for damages for mental pain and suffering caused by alleged negligence, carelessness and breach of contract. In this case, the acts complained of were that the father was told that his child, born in the hospital, was a girl, but later was told that the child was a boy. The court dismissed the action on the grounds that, in the absence of physical injury, the complaint was not sufficient to state a cause of action in tort. Also, it failed to state a cause of action for breach of contract.[5] Even though this action was dismissed, the fact that a legal action was brought will tend to make a busy nurse, who frequently handles inquiries concerning patients over the telephone or in person, attentive to both her replies and the person to whom they are addressed.

In one case, a mother being discharged from the hospital following childbirth was given an infant purported to be her own. Some time later the parents discovered that the nurse had given them the wrong baby. They brought the error to the hospital's attention and were given another child, who, the hospital stated, was their baby. The parents were denied a recovery of damages.[6] Although the court agreed that the action complained of was negligence, still, in the absence of proof of any physical suffering, an award was not permitted for mental suffering alone.

When an 89-year-old patient in a nursing home died from pneumonia caused by the ingestion of kerosene, a verdict against the nursing home for damages for his death was upheld.[7]

The parents of a boy recovered in excess of a quarter of a million dollars damages against a hospital for the negligence of the nurses which resulted in injuries to their child at birth.[8] Specifically, they charged that nurses in the hospital's delivery room in 1957 had delayed the baby's birth by pressing a towel against his head until an obstetrician arrived. As a result, they claimed, oxygen to the baby's brain was cut off; he is retarded and will require special care for life.

Hospital nurses were cleared in the death of a patient who died from pulmonary edema shortly after a blood transfusion was completed in a case in which the attending physician set the amount of blood to be administered at 1000 cc., started the procedure and set the stopcock at the desired rate of flow. The nurses kept the patient under observation for five to 15 minutes.[9]

Recently, the New York and California courts have allowed recovery of damages for mental anguish. In 1959, a patient collected $15,000 for cancer-phobia resulting from a physician's warning that a radiation burn might lead eventually to cancer. A California mother who was seven months pregnant when she saw an ice truck run over her small son was severely shocked, and received damages when the court said:

> No immutable rule calls for physical impact to justify recovery for emotional distress.[10]

However, in another suit against a doctor and hospital for psychic injury because of alleged erroneous diagnosis and treatment, the case was dismissed.[11] The allegedly erroneous diagnosis was that an arrested pulmonary tuberculosis condition had become active and that the germs were in the stomach and might have reached the intestine. The patient claimed he had undergone unnecessary chemotherapy. The patient was well at the time of trial, and the court felt that the doctor's error (if he was in error) was understandable, if not an error of judgment.

COMMON ACTS OF NEGLIGENCE

Let us look into some of the common acts of negligence.

Overlooked Sponges

One of the most common acts of negligence in surgical cases in the past has been the overlooked sponge. Either the nurse failed to make a check on the number of sponges or there was an error in her sponge count, and the surgeon closed the incision with a sponge or sponges left inside the patient. As a result, infections and delayed recoveries or even death ensued, and then there would be actions for damages for negligence.

In a California case in which a sponge was left in a patient and the surgeon neither counted the sponges nor required a sponge count by a nurse, the charitable hospital was held not liable for the acts of the nurses, since they were under the control of the surgeon. However, the surgeon was liable for the negligent act.[12]

On the other hand, in another case, an action was brought against a student nurse and others for damages for death of a patient. There a student nurse simply passed out sponges to a surgeon during the operation, but did not count sponges afterward. A supervising nurse was responsible for the sponge count at the conclusion of the operation. The supervising nurse reported that the sponge count was correct, when in fact a sponge had been left in the patient. The student nurse was held not liable, but the supervising nurse was held liable.[13]

Out of an award of $36,000, a scrub nurse and a circulating nurse had to pay $4000 apiece in a case in which a laparotomy sponge was left in a patient during abdominal surgery and they had reported the sponge count correct.[14] Since the surgeon had ordered the metal rings removed from the sponges, which was a safeguard provided by the employer, he became the nurses' special employer during the surgery and was liable with them.

A patient undergoing abdominal surgery and the removal of three moles sustained burns from the contact place of the "Bovie machine," which the physician had directed the nurse to prepare; the court ruled that there was sufficient evidence and that this was a question of fact on which a jury could find negligence.[15]

Burns

Along with missing sponges, at the head of the list of negligent acts frequently charged to nurses, are burns of one kind or another from hot water bottles, heating pads, inhalators, contact with steam pipes, radiators, scalding hot water, douches, sitz baths, sweat cabinets, and solutions which are either too hot or of improper concentration for the purpose used. A nurse, notwithstanding the stage of her training, may be liable for certain acts. It does not require a technical education to know that very hot objects burn persons. Consequently, if a student nurse with only a little professional education and training, or a practical nurse, were to fill a hot water bottle with excessively hot water and place it against an unconscious person, whereby he was burned, she would in all likelihood be deemed liable for such an act. In other words, it is questionable whether an ordinary nurse of similar training using due care in such circumstances would thus burn a patient with a hot water bottle; if not, the nurse who did burn a patient is liable for her failure to use that degree of care.

When a patient sustained a third degree burn because a surgeon placed a hot metal gag in her mouth during a tonsillectomy, a verdict in favor of the surgeon and instrument nurse but against the hospital was returned by the jury. According to testimony, it was the duty of the circulating nurse to have available a basin of water for cooling instruments after their sterilization and its negligent omission was the cause of the accident.[16]

A patient who was paralyzed and could not remove his pipe from his mouth safely and who had a speech impediment was left alone while smoking his pipe, which fell from his mouth, setting fire to the bed; as a result he was burned. He received a judgment against the hospital.[17] Nurses have a duty to protect the patient from any known danger.

The court ruled that the government was liable to the administratrix of the estate of an 83-year-old patient who was senile and generally *non compos mentis* and suffering from a possible cerebral vascular accident when he was burned while in the bathtub at an Army hospital.[18] The injuries were caused by the negligence of hospital employees in allowing scalding water to stand in the hot water pipe leading directly into the bathtub, and in the course of a struggle with the attendant assisting him from the tub, the patient had accidentally turned on the hot water.

A paying patient in a hospital conducted for profit by a municipality in Oklahoma recovered damages for injuries due to burns caused by a hot enema negligently administered by a registered nurse.[19]

In a case in Virginia, $13,000 damages were awarded to a woman patient for burns of tissue caused by negligence in injecting dye into a vein before taking x-rays and in applying a hot water bottle which resulted in a partial disability of the patient's arm and in physical and neurotic ailments that might never improve. The intern and nurse were held to be employees of the hospital and not independent contractors. Both were considered to be working directly under the hospital's supervision and control and acting on behalf of the hospital. The court distinguished no substantial difference in their relation to the patient.[20]

The hospital was not exempt from liability in an Oklahoma case in which a nurse burned a patient by placing an unguarded lamp globe on her body without direction, but while in the presence of a physician. In this case, the physician was working directly over the patient immediately after an operation, attempting to save her from heart failure. The emergency required all his attention, and it was necessary to leave the other details of postoperative care to the nurse.[21]

On the other hand, when a patient was instructed in the operation of an electric heating pad and he successfully operated it for three days, neither the nurse nor the hospital was held liable for burns caused by the pad when the patient went to sleep while the current was turned on. Here, the nurse could plead contributory negligence as a defense to the patient's claim.[22]

Actions of the pre-clinic student nurse have resulted in law suits. For example, an action was brought against a hospital to recover damages for injuries due to alleged negligence of such student nurse in giving a woman after childbirth a douche which, either because it contained an excessive quantity of bichloride of mercury or because it was too hot, burned her body.[23] The dismissal on the following day of the young woman of 18, who had entered training six months before, was part of the evidence. In this case, the question of the hospital's using due care in the selection of the nurse arose. The verdict was awarded for the patient.

When a nurse placed a steam vaporizer on the side of the bed where the bathroom was located and the patient tripped over it and was injured, the court held that negligence could be inferred from the nurse's failure to put the vaporizer on the opposite side of the bed.[24] The nurse is required to use reasonable judgment in carrying out a doctor's order.

Falls

Possibly next in frequency are suits for damages against nurses and hospitals by patients who have fallen out of bed and as a result suffered injuries. Sometimes the patient may be one who is allowed to get up, but who falls while getting out of a high hospital bed. Accidents of this kind often occur with elderly persons, those who have had sedatives, postoperative patients who have not fully recovered from anesthesia, blind persons, semiconscious persons or sufferers from dizziness.

Side rails and other restraints, when ordered, prevent or reduce the hazard of such falls. It would almost seem unnecessary to say that when an unconscious or partially conscious patient is returned to his bed after an operation, in the absence of a qualified attendant giving constant attention, the side rails should be put up immediately. Such a precautionary measure is at times neglected, and this in turn leads to falls, injuries, and law suits for resulting damages. In some hospitals, it is a routine to place side rails on the beds of all postoperative patients, irrational patients, and at night on the beds of all patients who are 60 or more years of age or under six years. In New York, it is considered an administrative act, and the hospital is liable if a nurse fails to carry out the instructions of a physician for using side rails as a precaution for the patient's protection from falling from bed.[25] Certainly delirious patients need side rails and constant care to prevent accidents.

If a pre-clinic student nurse is given the assignment of watching a patient, keeping him covered, and preventing him from falling out of bed, she could be held responsible for his injuries unless the patient became unmanageable. The reasoning here is that any adult of sound mind and body should be able to carry out such an assignment unless the patient is unmanageable.[26] If the nurse were a practical nurse in the circumstances just given, she too would be liable unless the patient was unmanageable. If the patient in such circumstances fell from the bed and was injured, the blame attached to the student or practical nurse would depend upon whether she had used such precaution as could be expected from an ordinary, reasonably prudent nurse with similar training in such circumstances.

As previously observed, the nurse will notice the split of authority on whether an institution is liable for the negligent acts of its employees. When a paying patient who was in a helpless condition fell from a chair through the negligence of the servants of a private hospital, the courts held that a cause of action was stated to recover damages from the hospital.[27] In another case, in which, in the absence of her nurses, a patient jumped to her death, a charitable hospital in Maine was not held liable for the neglect of its servants on the grounds that such a charitable institution is immune from liability.[28]

When a nurse attending a mother during labor negligently failed to summon an intern in sufficient time for delivery, and the resident seemingly misunderstood the urgency of the call, the baby suffered a birth injury, and the parents recovered substantial damages on behalf of the infant girl.[29]

When a restless elderly woman who was suffering from pain and shock following injuries was placed in a hospital bed with a side rail only on the side of the bed away from the wall, and she fell from the bed sustaining injuries, a judgment for the hospital was reversed.[30]

A substantial verdict was rendered in behalf of a patient known to have neurological problems who fell and sustained serious injuries when she was unattended and became dizzy in the hallway enroute from the bathroom during the night.[31]

A verdict for damages was reversed in a case in which a patient failed to show that a fall from the examining table in the emergency room of the hospital was due to the negligence of the hospital.[32] The patient had been brought to the emergency room following a heart attack. She could not prove that she had been unconscious when left unattended. There was some evidence that she was conscious, and she had been secured to the table by a belt and the side rails of the table had been raised.

An award of $115,000 to the widow for the wrongful death of her husband was not excessive in a case in which the hospital's technicians had left the patient alone on an x-ray table while he was in a sleepy, tired, and dazed condition and under the influence of drugs.[33] The court held that they should have foreseen that the patient, who was complaining of nausea, would attempt to go to the bathroom and would likely injure himself in so doing because of the effect of the drugs.

A judgment for a patient for injuries sustained when he fell from bed was affirmed for a 73-year-old man who suffered a heart attack and was taken to the defendant hospital. His daughter testified that he was "dazed" and "didn't know where he was."[34] The court held that the jury could find the patient's conduct was a result of drugs or a mental condition caused by the heart attack and not a result of the patient's conscious volition.

How long a patient may be safely left alone by the nurses depends on the facts of each case. When a woman was given three grains of Tuinol, Phenergan and 50 mg. of Demerol and Scopolamine before delivery and 2 cc. of 2 x Duladumone afterward, and was left alone in a private room for an hour and five minutes, during which time she fell out of bed and was injured, the court took the view that the patient was not alert due to heavy sedation and was not properly attended.[35]

If errors in drug distribution are to be avoided, nursing service, pharmacists and hospital administration must cooperate on a sound policy to eliminate errors and must adhere to it.[36]

Failure to Observe and Take Appropriate Action

Nurses who disregard a mother's pleas and who fail to observe and evaluate a child's condition and secure timely medical assistance may make the hospital liable for actionable negligence.[37] There was testimony that the 13-year-old rheumatic fever patient was coughing almost constantly, that her nails turned blue and that her heart pounded until the mattress shook over a six-hour period, while the distraught mother's pleas for help brought little except personal reprimands. Eventually, when the supervisor of nurses found the mother crying in a hallway and hurried to the child's room, the physician in charge of the patient was summoned. Despite intensive care and the efforts of the doctor and special duty nurses, the child died the following day.

A college football player sustained a broken leg. It was placed in a cast at a community hospital. The foot became cold two days later and there was a foul smell in the room for two weeks, and eventually the leg had to be amputated at a medical center to which the patient was transferred. He recovered damages.[38] Not long after the cast was applied, the patient complained of pain, and his toes were swollen and became dark. The cast was cut several times, and in so doing, the leg was also cut. After two weeks the patient was transferred to a medical center. The community hospital was held liable under *respondeat superior* because the nurses either did not observe or at least failed to report patient problems that were overlooked or not thought to be significant by the doctor. The physician himself settled out of court; he had no specialty training and had not secured consultation.

When a mother, following delivery of her daughter, died of a hemorrhage from a laceration of the cervix, and a nurse did not take her pulse, blood pressure, temperature or respiration or call her doctor, even though she was aware that the bleeding was more than normal postpartum flow and in time that the patient's condition was critical, the higher court reversed a verdict in favor of the nurse, hospital and physician.[39] The court said:

> We are satisfied that the evidence was sufficient to support a finding that the nurses, Lee and Kiese, were negligent. . . . Conceding that Dr. Ashley was negligent, still if nurse Lee had called

the doctor at 10:30 P.M., when she was aware the condition of the patient was critical, who can say the same result would have occurred.

Wrong Medicines, Wrong Dosage, Wrong Concentration

Another group of common negligent acts includes wrong medicines, wrong dosage, wrong concentration of the proper medicine, misreading labels, neglecting to check labels, administering medicine to the wrong person, and similar errors.

The parents of an infant daughter in a wrongful death action recovered damages from a nurse and doctor for her accidental death due to an overdose of digitalis. With respect to the nurse, the court said:

> As laudable as her intentions are conceded to have been on the occasion in question, her unfamiliarity with the drug was a contributing factor in the child's death. In this regard we are of the opinion that she was negligent in attempting to administer a drug with which she was not familiar. . . . Not only was Mrs. Evans unfamiliar with the medicine in question but she also violated what has been shown to be a rule generally practiced by the members of the nursing profession in the community and which rule, we might add, strikes us as being most reasonable and prudent, namely, the practice of calling the prescribing physician when in doubt about an order for medication.[40]

The patient who became violently ill as a result of a licensed practical nurse's mistakenly administering internally the potassium permanganate pill meant for external use, could not recover damages from a charitable hospital where the nurse had completed a prescribed course for vocational nurses, had received a license from the state to practice nursing and had been practicing continuously for over three years.[41]

A judgment for $700 was affirmed against a hospital and nurse for injuries sustained when the nurse put hydrochloric acid in the patient's nose instead of nose drops.[42]

A passenger on a bus, injured when the bus driver lost consciousness and the bus struck a telephone pole, recovered a substantial sum from the bus company and driver, whose lapse of consciousness was attributed to the side effects of the medicine, Pyribenzamine, which his doctor had prescribed.[43] The patient had been given no warning of the side effects of the drug and had taken his first pill on the morning of the accident. The value of instructing patients who are to take their own medications – the teaching function of nursing as well as that of physicians – seems apparent.

When the parents of an infant sued a physician and an assistant physician for crippling damage to the infant's leg as the result of a student nurse's erroneously injecting a drug into the muscles of the infant's buttocks, the physicians settled out of court for $10,000.[44] The student nurse ignored a warning on the ampule that the drug was for intravenous use only.

The court of appeals ruled that the allegation of a child's mother that the amount of Demerol given the child following surgery was greater than the amount the nurse charted was sufficient to raise an issue of fact.[45] The child had died following an injection of Demerol administered after a tonsillectomy and circumcision.

When a paying patient sued a county in Idaho for damages for an injury caused by the wrong solution administered by a nurse employed by the hospital, the patient was allowed to recover from the county. In this instance, the nurse negligently supplied boric acid solution for injection in the patient's thigh instead of the saline solution requested.[46] In the majority of states, a person may not sue the government or a political subdivision of the state government without its consent in the absence of an express statutory provision.

In Oklahoma, a patient brought suit for damages for injuries caused by a nurse who did not follow the physician's directions in administering a hypodermic injection into the patient's hips instead of her arms. Abscesses resulted. However, when it was not shown that similar injuries would not have followed an injection in the patient's arms, the court held that as a matter of law the negligence of the nurse was not the proximate cause of the injuries.[47] However, the case serves to illustrate the point that the nurse should carry out the doctor's orders. Had this nurse carried out the doctor's orders as given, she would have eliminated this accusation of negligence and also the time, trouble and money involved in the court action.

Twenty thousand dollars was awarded to a patient who sustained a permanent foot drop and atrophy of the calf of his leg as the result of a nurse's negligently placing an injection in the wrong area of his buttock.[48]

In a case in which a nurse negligently administered a solution of 10 per cent sodium hydroxide instead of an 85 per cent saline solution as part of a gastric analysis, causing serious injuries and some permanent disability, the patient was awarded $162,500 damages.[49]

A hospital patient received an injection of fluid for a diagnostic test from a nurse, and thereafter infection in her arm followed by thrombophlebitis occurred. She recovered damages on the doctrine of *res ipsa loquitur,* since the procedure was under the hospital's control and there was some evidence of failure to maintain sterility.[50]

Administration of Blood by Nurses

The question frequently arises as to whether a registered professional nurse who has had adequate instruction and experience may start and administer blood under the direction of a physician. It is pertinent to remind nurses of what Emanuel Hayt has said repeatedly:

> There is probably no biologic product in medical therapy that carries with it more possible sources of dangerous error than blood.[51]

When hospital policy or the law does not preclude the nurse from doing some procedure, and when she has had adequate instruction and experience, it is probably the general rule that she can do the procedure under the direction and supervision of a duly licensed physician.

At the same time, it is pointed out that what a registered professional nurse may do legally and what it is desirable for her to do may be quite different matters. With respect to cut-downs, except in a dire emergency when no physician is available, the nurse should not make an incision to reach a vein.[52]

The patient's name and hospital number should be attached to each unit of blood, and the information should be carefully verified with the patient's identification armband. During the transfusion, the patient should be observed carefully; if there are any untoward symptoms, reactions or complaints by the patient, the transfusion should be stopped and the physician notified and further direction requested. It is an obligation of the nurse to make certain that every requisition for blood has the patient's complete name and hospital number.[53]

A patient who was recovering from surgery was informed by a hospital nurse and intern that she was to have a blood transfusion. The intern started the transfusion and she suffered a reaction to it, followed by other ills. The transfusion had not been ordered for her by the attending physician, and the hospital was held liable.[54] The court went on to say that the patient was entitled to be protected from trespass and assault if it could be reasonably anticipated, and that the wrongs were due to the very person whom the hospital employed to care for patients.

In an action against a blood bank by a hospital patient for breach of implied warranty — the patient contracted hepatitis after she received blood transfusions — the judgment was in favor of the defendant.[55] Furnishing blood to a patient for a transfusion charged for by the hospital does not constitute a sale, and the patient cannot recover for breach of implied warranty of its fitness for use.

Failure to Communicate

Three days after a caesarean section, a patient complained of soreness in her jaw and in opening her mouth. Although a nurse and a resident gave her several medications, they did not notify the physician of her complaint. When her physician finally discovered the patient's symptoms on a visit, he administered tetanus antitoxin and remained with her until her death that night. The appellate court dismissed the charge against the physician and affirmed a judgment that the hospital was liable for the failure of its employees to give timely notification to the doctor of the patient's condition.[56]

Failure to Exercise Reasonable Judgment

A young married woman received an award of damages for injuries and permanent scarring in a case in which a nurse did not discontinue an injection of saline solution into the patient's breasts for hypodermoclysis treatment after it became evident that it was adversely affecting the unconscious patient.[57] The nurse who carries out any medical order must exercise reasonable judgment. When there are changes in the patient's condition which would indicate some change in therapy, she is expected to communicate with the physician for modification or confirmation of his written orders. If he is not available, she must communicate with another physician.

Defects in Apparatus

Defects in apparatus may cause injury. If the defects are obvious, the nurse is thereby warned against using the equipment, but the nurse cannot be held responsible for knowing hidden defects in equipment. A hospital which furnishes defective equipment is liable to the patient who is injured by the same.[58] If a nurse uses obviously defective equipment, she will be liable to a patient for injuries caused by the same. A nurse's training and experience familiarize her with supplies and equipment which are of an acceptable standard.

The danger of infection from the use of an unsterile needle is a matter of common knowledge. A nurse's use of an unsterile needle would in all probability be considered negligent. In cases involving physicians, the courts have so held.[59]

An older hospital visitor, who was injured when the chair she sat in collapsed, recovered damages from the hospital because no one made regular inspections in order to discover and repair defective conditions.[60]

Errors Due to Family Assistance in Patient Care

Although parents, spouses, relatives and friends who assist in caring for a patient may be psychologically and emotionally comforting, the nurse must remember that they may complicate the liability problem. When an accident occurs, certain questions inevitably arise, such as whether the act done by the relative was one which should have been done by a nurse. In the matter of negligence, it is possible for a relative as well as a nurse to be negligent. If the patient is injured as a result of the relative's negligence, may he recover damages from the hospital? Relatives concerned with the patient's comfort may do things contrary to the doctor's orders — matters of diet, turning and coughing patients, and self-help as a part of rehabilitation are examples of areas in which relatives may, at times, undo a part of the plan of therapy. In any event, rules for relatives should be reviewed by the hospital or agency legal counsel.[61]

Abandonment

In one case, a nurse left a baby alone, and the infant crawled to an unprotected radiator and was burned. In another case, a nurse left the room suddenly in the course of giving a patient a bath and left her uncovered on a raw, cold morning for an hour, with the result that the patient got pneumonia. In both instances, the nurse's action was considered negligent.

When a patient is injured, or his illness is aggravated and extended by negligent acts of the nurse, the nurse makes herself liable for suit for damages not only for the expenses of a longer stay in the hospital, but also for the extra time (and therefore money) lost by the patient's being away from his job.

Loss of or Damage to Patient's Property

A nurse may be accused of negligence in the care of a patient's property. Possibly the item most frequently involved is the patient's dentures. In the course of her training, each nurse has been taught some simple but effective method of handling dentures to prevent damage and loss, such as placing them in a transparent container or container conspicuously and specifically labeled for the purpose. And it is a wise nurse who adheres to such a practice in her work. However, if a denture is wrapped in a piece of tissue or paper towel, it is easy to understand how such an unlabeled, crumpled handful of (apparently) trash may subsequently be thrown out. Or, the denture may be damaged if it is placed where a heavy tray or other heavy object may be placed on it. In some modern dentures, the plastic used will crack if subjected to extremes of heat and cold.

A nurse's liability for the negligent loss of or damage to a patient's property is based upon her duty as a person, trained or untrained, to act as a reasonable and ordinary prudent person. Since in giving nursing care to patients a nurse customarily must from time to time handle the patients' various personal belongings, placing them in drawers and lockers provided therefor, she must use reasonable care in so doing. Not only is the nurse personally liable for her acts of negligence in regard to a patient's property, but if she is an employee or agent she may render her employer liable as well.

Definition of bailment. At this point, it should be mentioned that when a patient deposits personal property, such as money, rings, or watches, with another, a bailment is created. The person who deposits the property is a "bailor," and the person with whom the property is deposited is a "bailee." A bailment is a contract in which property is deposited for keeping and is to be delivered at a certain time to the bailor on his order and payment made for such service. In a typical hospital situation, however, the depositing of a patient's property with the hospital or a nurse represents a gratuitous type of bailment, whereby the nurse or hospital agrees to care for such property. In this case, if the patient's property is injured or lost, there is an action for damages for negligence. As previously discussed, once a person undertakes to do an act or give a service, he must use due care.

Infections

Nurses, especially through their adherence (or lack of it) to aseptic technique, may be a factor in infections or cross-infections. Certainly, when an infection can be prevented by ordinary, reasonable care, nurses are bound to use such care, and if they fail to do so they may be held liable for damages.

Since the professional nurse is responsible for supervising the safety and security of the patient, she must be concerned with his environment.[62] In an action against an infirmary and a doctor to recover damages for the death of a daughter who died from lockjaw following an appendectomy, evidence as to the matters of the cleanliness of the floor, cleaning by sweeping with a broom (causing dust) rather than using a mop, improper sterilization of instruments, insufficient heating of the rooms in which the patient was placed and improper care of the wound following the operation were held admissible.[63] Postoperative wound infection may be due to negligence in cleaning the floors and improper or inadequate sterilization of equipment. Infection may be due to cross-contamination. Damages in a malpractice action for the death of a 12-day-old child were awarded in a case in which the nurse negligently permitted the infant to become infected with impetigo.[64] The nurse erroneously gave the baby's mother another infant, who was suffering from impetigo, to nurse; thereafter her own baby became infected with impetigo.

In a suit brought by a woman to recover damages for an infection following childbirth, the court held that she was entitled to damages because there was evidence that medical students subjected her to rectal and vaginal examinations after taking their hands from their pockets.[65] Justice Dooling said:

> We will likewise take judicial notice of the danger of infection to a woman about to give birth to a child from a vaginal examination performed with unsterile hands.

The hospital was held responsible for the death of a baby from miliary tuberculosis shortly after its birth who was cared for in the nursery by a nurse with tuberculosis.[66] The parents of the baby were not tubercular. The nurse had a cough, yet those who had a duty to report her condition apparently did not; it was negligence to allow her to work.

However, in another case, damages for the infection of a newborn were sought in an action for negligence in admitting to the hospital the mother of an infant immediately prior to the birth of the infant during the course of an infection affecting infants in the hospital without notice thereof to the expectant mother. The court ruled that the record failed to show any actionable negligence on the part of the hospital.[67]

In a malpractice action against a plastic surgeon, in which the plaintiff's face was worse than when she started due to infection following an operation to remove a scar, the court ruled that there was no presumption of negligence, because of the fact that infection occurs at the site of treatment.[68]

Awards to parents and their newborn infant for injuries suffered from *Staphylococcus aureus* infection were set aside by the state supreme court. The evidence permitted the jury to find that the newborn baby contracted *Staphylococcus aureus* infection while in the hospital and that the baby's father and mother contracted it as a result, but there was insufficient evidence of negligence by the hospital in caring for the infant.[69]

A patient did recover in excess of $67,000 damages for injuries resulting from a staphylococcus infection contracted in a hospital, and his wife recovered consequential damages when there was evidence that the hospital nursing staff touched the patient's roommate, who had a boil discharging pus, and then touched the plaintiff without observing the sterile techniques prescribed by the hospital in cases in which infection is suspected.[70] When a culture of the roommate's drainage showed it to have been caused by *Staphylococcus aureus*, he was removed to an isolation room. However, the staphylococcus infection penetrated the hip joint of the patient, who was undergoing hip surgery as a result of an automobile accident; this necessitated a second operation, in which the patient's hip was fused in a nearly immobile position. The lack of sterile technique in caring for these two patients, the possibility that mass transfers of germs could have occurred and the time between the discharge of pus from the roommate's boil and the subsequent drainage from the patient's hip were enough to spell out the cause of the plaintiff's infection.

In some situations, evidence of what occurred is inaccessible to the injured person. However, the law has a rule known as *res ipsa loquitur*, or "the thing speaks for itself," which may be applied to certain negligence cases. Three conditions are necessary before this rule may be applied: (1) that in the ordinary course of affairs the accident would not have occurred if reasonable care were used, (2) that the thing that caused the accident was under the exclusive control of the defendant, and (3) that the plaintiff did not contribute to the occurrence of the accident.[71] When the plaintiff proves that these conditions exist, it is regarded in some states as circumstantial evidence of negligence, which judge or jury may accept or reject, while in other states it is held to create a presumption of negligence.

Thus, judgment was entered for the parents who sued a hospital and physicians to recover damages for malpractice resulting in the loss of a 2-day-old boy's glans penis as a result of circumcision.[72] Judgment was also affirmed for a plaintiff who developed fever and chills and infection of the urinary passages after a cystoscopic examination.[73] However, in an action to recover damages for a burn allegedly caused by the application of hot water bottles during a surgical procedure, the verdict was in favor of the doctor and hospital, as there was evidence that the injury might have resulted from other causes not attributable to any negligence on the part of the defendants.[74]

More recently, the parents of a baby girl born prematurely at a U.S. Naval hospital recovered damages for her injuries and deformity as a result of osteomyelitis in the hips caused by a staphylococcus infection. One nurse in the nursery had a positive nose culture for staphylococcus, and it was shown that she did not receive a physical examination when reporting on duty at this hospital, although she had had one shortly before leaving her previous post of duty.[75]

MALPRACTICE AS CAUSE FOR DAMAGES

Malpractice in the usual sense implies the idea of improper or unskillful care of a patient by a nurse. In any cause of action brought for damages in civil courts, as distinguished from causes of action in criminal courts, no difference is made between willfulness and negligence from the point of view of either damages or culpability. The degree of culpability is often vital in a criminal case. There is no actionable negligence, in other words no suit for malpractice, unless there is a duty on the defendant to protect the plaintiff from harm which might come from the defendant's unskilled or careless actions, a violation of such duty, and a resultant injury to the plaintiff which can be traced to breach of duty.[76]

Malpractice vs. Negligence

Some authorities believe that the differences between negligence and malpractice are not too well distinguished, and that it is preferable to consider malpractice synonymous with professional negligence. In a California case, the court defined malpractice in relation to a nurse:

> Malpractice is the neglect of a physician or nurse to apply that degree of skill and learning in treating and nursing a patient which is customarily applied in treating and caring for the sick or wounded similarly suffering in the same community.[77]

On the other hand, it would seem that malpractice also denotes a stepping beyond one's authority with serious consequences.

Malpractice Acts

Giving general anesthetics. It has sometimes been held that it is illegal for a nurse to give general anesthetics. A licensed and registered nurse employed by a hospital in California who administered general anesthetics in connection with operations under the direction of a surgeon and his assistants was held not to be engaged in illegal "practice of medicine" in violation of the Medical Practice Act. It was ruled that the nurse was not "diagnosing or prescribing" while assisting in surgery. Moreover, the nurse's activities were under control of the surgeons.[78] When done under the supervision of a physician, the giving of general anesthetics may be considered a professional nursing function.

Failure to exercise due care and reasonableness. In a malpractice suit against a hospital, a registered nurse and a physician, it was alleged that the surgeon was operating to remove a cyst from the wall of an abdomen. He ordered the preparation of a one per cent procaine solution. A solution of formaldehyde was negligently prepared in its place and handed to him by the nurse. The court held that the surgeon was allowed to rely on the skill and care of trained nurses and similar persons. The nurse was held liable by the court on the grounds that she did not read the label on the formaldehyde bottle and because she knew that the physician was going to use the solution he had ordered to produce local anesthesia on the patient.[79] In short, a nurse as a professionally trained person must exercise all the due care and reasonableness associated with the training of members of her profession. In the case cited, in which the nurse was aware of the purpose for which the solution was to be used, and by training knew, or should have known, the properties of formaldehyde and procaine, she was not justified in unquestioningly heeding the surgeon's order even if she understood him to say formaldehyde instead of Novocain. On the other hand, if she handed the surgeon a syringe full of a drug without reading and checking the label, she was not using the due care of an ordinary reasonable and prudent professional registered nurse under similar circumstances.

In the case which follows, a physician was sued for alleged negligence of his nurse, but held not liable. The nurse took out of a medicine cabinet a bottle labeled "silver nitrate," the percentage of which was illegible. Knowing that a solution of only one per cent (customarily used in a newborn's eyes) was usually kept there, she filled a dropper and instilled it while the doctor held open the infant's eyes. It was in fact a 30 per cent solution and impaired the infant's vision.[80] Again, the nurse is reminded that customarily in her training, she is taught to read the label three times on a medicine container and to use no medicine from a container the label of which is illegible. The wisdom of adhering to such training and standard of care is obvious.

In an action for damages against an Indiana private hospital, the plaintiff sued because of malpractice in diagnosis and treatment of injury of the patient's left hip. The owner or proprieter of the hospital, which is operated for private gain and not for charity, was liable for the injury sustained by the patient due to the negligence of nurses or other employees.[81]

The plaintiff in another case sued a hospital and doctors for the death of a child as a result of what was claimed to be malpractice in permitting a baby to become infected with impetigo and negligence in treating the infection and in discharging the plaintiff's wife and baby while the infant was still suffering with impetigo. A judgment of $6000 was awarded for the death of the 12-day-old baby.[82] Since nurses care for newborn infants, and since such nursing service is frequently given to babies in a nursery situation at hospitals, the responsibility, duty, failure and liability of a nurse are apparent.

New Rule in Medical Malpractice

Ever since the *Small v. Howard*[83] case some 90 years ago, in which the court ruled that a village practitioner would be required to have only knowledge and skills of other practitioners of ordinary ability and skill in "similar localities, with opportunities for no larger experience," the community test of malpractice has been generally applied as the legal standard for physicians, nurses and others. When the court held the physician guilty of malpractice in making a mistake in diagnosis and medical mismanagement in the care of a child born of parents with Rh factor blood incompatibility, it said:

> To fasten liability in a malpractice case, the patient must prove by a preponderence of evidence the recognized standard of medical care in the community, and that the physician being sued departed from that standard in treating the patient.[84]

Recently, however, the *Brune v. Belinkoff* decision has overruled this precedent.[85] In this new decision, the court required the anesthesiologist practicing in a smaller city to follow a general standard of care applicable to all specialists in his field. Furthermore, the

court stated that it would apply the same rule to general practitioners. This decision should help the regional medical programs to
attain the goal of bringing the latest and best in modern health care
to practitioners in all areas of the country.

Professional Liability Insurance Coverage by Employer

As James has pointed out, many nurses erroneously assume that
they are protected by their hospital's professional liability policies,
yet only about 2 per cent of the hospitals in the United States insure
their employees under a paramedical endorsement.[86] When the hospital or other employer tells the nurse she is "covered" by his insurance, she would do well to ask for a certificate of insurance. A
nurse needs her own policy, since she may be sued individually as
well as along with her employer and also because when the employer
has to pay damages, the insurance company may seek subrogation
(restitution) from the nurse. For example, an insurance company filed
a subrogation for $10,000 against an L.P.N. who paid $400 down and
then faced a long period of indebtedness.[87]

Nurses should note that the authority who states that hospitals
win 92 per cent of the cases tried stresses the importance of reviewing
nurses' notes and incident reports.[88]

Even if a hospital does protect its employees with a professional
liability policy, the nurse should realize that in a number of instances
she will be carrying out duties under the direction or supervision of a
physician or surgeon and will be considered temporarily as his special
employee. Now, although the physician or surgeon likely carries
malpractice insurance that covers him and any person for whom he is
legally liable, it would not cover the individual liability of such an
employee (and an employee is always personally liable to suit for his
own negligence). It is infrequent that the physician's liability policy
protects the nurse; hence her own individual liability policy is
desirable.

The industrial nurse will find that industry seldom has professional liability insurance, and that if they do, her personal liability is
not included. Since the industrial nurse works more on her own, and
the physician is not so readily available in case of need, she needs to
consider seriously the need for her own professional liability
coverage.

Nurse's Own Professional Liability Insurance

When a nurse does plan to secure liability insurance, she should
shop for a policy that will best protect her. Quite often nursing
organizations offer the nurse a liability insurance policy through the

group. Heinz cites the following statement from the policy of a major company as one that offers the nurse good protection:

> To pay all loss by reason of the liability imposed by law upon the insured for damages on account of professional services rendered or which should have been rendered by the insured or any assistant to the insured during the term of this policy including the dispensing of drugs or medicine or any counter-claims in suit brought by the insured to collect fees providing such damages are claimed under any of the foregoing.[89]

SOME PRECAUTIONS TO OBSERVE

The nurse must learn the basic facts of her profession; she must learn to observe, to evaluate, and to judge a patient's condition. In addition, she must learn to perform her duties with at least the care of the ordinary, reasonable and prudent nurse in those particular circumstances. She must realize that she is personally responsible for her own wrongful or negligent acts and that as an employee or agent she may render her employer liable.

If in doubt about a written order from a physician, the nurse should make sure that she understands it before attempting to carry it out. The situation is somewhat like the story of the bad egg; if there is any doubt about it, there is no doubt about it. She should secure an interpretation or verification of the order if it is not clear. There are tactful ways of securing explanations.

If, in pursuit of her nursing assignment, a nurse notices an adverse effect of a medicine the doctor has ordered administered to a patient, she should not continue to carry out orders blindly, but should report adverse effects immediately and request further orders. Part of the nurse's duty is to observe symptoms and reactions and report them.

A nurse, the same as any other person in the course of everyday human activities, may render medical care in an emergency, and in so doing she would not be liable for violating medical practice acts.

A nurse is not authorized to give medical opinions either before a case is brought up in court or in testimony at a trial. Like any other witness on the stand, a nurse may state what she has seen, heard or done.[90]

We have mentioned before the fact that insurance is available for the protection of the nurse. Some authorities believe that all registered nurses should carry malpractice insurance to cover the cost of expert legal protection and to pay possible claims for damages.

COMMENT

It is the responsibility of the nurse to learn her profession. In a practical situation, learning, knowledge and skills that are not possessed cannot be applied. In her classes in nursing education, the nurse learns what is expected of her in her profession. She learns the standards and scope of her duties and what reasonable care means. The nurse learns the distinction between medical practice and the practice of nursing; the professions are closely linked together, yet they are separate professions.

Because the nurse often renders bedside care important to the patient's comfort, a patient may ask her what she thinks is the matter in a given case. An unwary nurse might state her opinions and make a diagnosis. It is obvious that quotations to doctors of what she said could lead to trouble. Early in her career it is wise for the nurse to develop a firm habit of not discussing with a patient his ailments, the various types of treatment, or various doctors. When a patient desires more information about his condition, it is prudent for a nurse to suggest that the patient consult his doctor. If a nurse deports herself with discretion, she will not only avoid legal troubles arising from wrongful practice of medicine, but she will also make an important contribution to lessening malpractice suits against physicians and surgeons.

REFERENCES

1. Prosser: *Torts* (Hornbook, 1964) § 35, 36. Cf. *Restatement, Torts,* § 281 Palsgraf v. Long Island R. Co., 248 N.Y. 339, 162 N.E. 99, 59 A.L.R. 1263 (1928)
2. Napier v. Greenzweig, 256 Fed. 196 (2d Cir., 1919); Forthofer v. Arnold, 60 Ohio App. 436, 21 N.E. 2d 869 (1938)
3. Rodgers v. Kline, 56 Miss. 808, 31 Am. Rep. 389 (1879)
4. Regan: *Doctor and Patient and the Law,* 3rd ed. 1956, p. 493
5. Kaufman v. Israel Zion Hospital, 183 Misc. 714, 51 N.Y.S. 2d 412 (1944)
6. Espinosa v. Beverly Hospital *et al.,* 249 P. 2d 843 (Calif., 1953)
7. Granite Home v. Schwartz, 364 S.W. 2d 309 (Ark. 1963)
8. Deutsch v. Doctors Hospital, *The AMA News,* Oct. 4, 1965, p. 2
9. Powell v. Fidelity & Casualty Co. of New York, 185 So. 2d 324 (1966)
10. Amaya v. Home Ice, Fuel & Supply Co., 23 Cal. Rptr. 131 (1962)
11. Kraus v. Spielberg and Jewish Hospital of Brooklyn, 37 Misc. 2d 519, 236 N.Y.S. 2d 143 (1962)
12. Armstrong v. Wallace 8 Cal. App. 2d 429, 37 P 2d 467, 47 P 2d 740 (1935)
13. Piper v. Epstein, 326 Ill. App. 400, 62 N.E. 2d 139 (1945)
14. Martin v. Perth Amboy Hospital *et al.,* 1969 CCH Neg. 4385 (N.J.)
15. Monk v. Doctors Hospital *et al.,* 1968 CCH Neg. 3908 (Dist. of Col.)
16. Quinby v. Morrow *et al.,* 340 F 2d 584 (U.S. Ct. of Appeals, 2nd Cir., Vt., 1965)
17. Hospital Authority of St. Mary's v. Eason, 148 S.E. 2d 499 (Ga., 1966)
18. Kopa v. United States, 236 F. Supp. 189 (D.C. Hawaii, 1964)
19. City of Shawnee v. Roush, 101 Okla. 60, 223 Pac. 354 (1924); *Hospitals,* X, 82-3 (Feb., 1936)
20. Stuart Circle Hospital Corporation v. Curry, 173 Va. 136, 3 S.E. 2d 153 (1939)
21. Flower Hospital v. Hart, 178 Okla. 447, 62 P. 2d 1248 (1936); *Hospitals,* XI, 106 (Apr., 1937)
22. Dittert v. Fischer, 148 Ore. 366, 36 P 2d 592 (1934); *Hospitals,* XIII, 99 (Feb., 1939)
23. Mills v. Richardson, 126 Me. 244, 137 Atl. 689 (1927)
24. Clark v. Piedmont Hospital, 117 Ga. App. 875, 162 S.E. 2d 418 (Ga. Ct. of Appeals, 1968)
25. Gordon, Adm. v. Harbor Hospital, Inc., 275 App. Div. 1047, 92 N.Y.S. 2d 1010, (1949)

26. Medicolegal abstract, Student Nurse: Patient Fell from Bed. *J.A.M.A.*, Bul. 115, No. 18, p. 1574, Nov., 1940
27. Robertson v. Executive Committee of Baptist Convention, 55 Ga. App. 469, 190 S.E. 432 (1937)
28. Jensen v. Maine Eye and Ear Infirmary, 107 Me. 408, 78 Atl. 898, 33 L.R.A. (N.S.) 141 (1910)
29. Garfield Memorial Hospital v. Marshall, 204 F. 2d 721 (U.S. Ct. of Appeals, D.C., 1953)
30. Strickland v. Bradford County Hospital, 196 So. 2d 765 (Fla., 1967)
31. Cardamon v. Iowa Lutheran Hospital, 128 N.W. 2d 226 (Iowa, 1964) Regan, William A.: Hospital Negligence Cases in the Court. *Hospital Progress,* 42:62-63, 128, June, 1961
32. South Broward Hospital District v. Schmitt, 172 So. 2d 12, cert. dism., 174 So. 2d 726 (Fla., 1965)
33. Hospital Authority of Hall County v. Adams, 110 Ga. App. 848, 140 S.E. 139 (1964)
34. Rhodes v. Moore *et al.,* 239 Ore. 454, 398 P. 2d 189 (1965)
35. Vick v. Methodist Evangelical Hosp., 1966 CCH Neg. 273 (Ky. 1966).
36. Regan, William A.: Where Legal Responsibilities Lie. *Hospitals,* 42: 55-58, Dec. 1, 1968
37. Duling v. Bluefield Sanitarium, Inc., 149 W. Va. 467, 142 N.E. 2d 754 (1965)
38. Darling v. Charleston Memorial Hospital, 211 N.E. 253 (W. Va., 1965); *Regan Report on Nursing Law* 5 (9) 3, Feb., 1965; Hershey, Nathan: Hospital's Expanding Responsibility. *Am. J. Nursing,* 66: 1546-7, July, 1966
39. Goff v. Buchanan Hospital, 333 P. 2d 29 (Cal. App., 1959); Parker, Leo T.: Liable for Negligence of Nurse. *Hosp. Topics,* 37:60-61, Dec., 1959
40. Norton v. Argonaut Insurance Co., 144 So. 2d 249 (Ct. of Appeals, La., 1962)
41. Penaloza v. Baptist Memorial Hospital, 304 S.W. 2d 203 (Tex., 1957)
42. Neel v. San Antonio Community Hospital, 1 Cal. Rptr. 313 (1959)
43. Kaiser v. Suburban Transportation System, 398 P. 2d 14, Amended 401 P. 2d 350 (Wash., 1965)
44. O'Neil v. Glen Falls Indemnity Co., 35 Am. Law Rep. 452, 310 Fed. 2d 165 (U.S. Ct. of Appeals, 8th Cir., 1962)
45. Ward v. Henderson *et al.,* 110 Ga. App. 780; 140 S.E. 2d 92, 142 S.E. 2d 244, 143 S.E. 2d 44 (Ga., 1965)
46. Henderson v. Twin Falls County, 56 Idaho 124, 50 P. 2d 597, Aff'm., 80 P. 2d 801 (1938)
47. Masonic Hospital Assoc. of Payne County v. Taggart, 171 Okla. 563, 43 P. 2d 142 (1935)
48. Wilmington General Hospital v. Nichols, 210 A. 2d 861 (Del., 1965). See also Regan, William A.: Nursing Policy and Hypodermic Injections. *Regan Report on Nursing Law,* 6 (2) 1, July, 1965
49. Gault v. Poor Sisters and St. Joseph Hospital, 1967 CCH Neg. Cases 1223
50. Southern Florida San. v. Hodge, 215 So. 2d 753 (Fla. 1968)
51. Hayt, Emanuel, *et al.: Law of Hospital and Nurse.* New York, Hospital Textbook Co., 1958, p. 198
52. Op. Atty. Gen. 368 (N.Y. 1942)
53. Champer, James: Historical and Legal Aspects of Blood Transfusions. *Hosp. Mgt.* 85:50, Feb., 1958
54. Necolayff v. Genesee Hospital, 61 N.Y.S. 2d 832, 270 App. Div. 648, Aff'm. 296 N.Y. 936, 73 N.E. 2d 117 (1947)
55. Whitehurst v. American National Red Cross, 1 Az. App. Rep. 326, 402 P. 2d 584 (1965)
56. Garafola v. Maimonides Hospital of Brooklyn *et al.,* 253 N.Y.S. 2d 856, Aff'd. 279 N.Y.S. 2d 523, 226 N.E. 311 (1967)
57. Parrish v. Clark, 107 Fla. 598, 145 So. 848 (1933)
58. Woodhouse v. Knickerbocker Hospital, 39 N.Y.S. 2d 671, Aff'm. 43 N.Y.S. 2d 518 (1943)
59. Clemens v. Smith, 170 Ore. 400, 134 P. 2d 424 (1943)
60. Dwyer v. Jackson, 20 Wis. 2d 318, 121 N.W. 2d 881 (1903)
61. Regan, William A.: Family Care No Substitute for RN Service. *Regan Report on Nursing Law,* 5(6)1, Nov., 1964

62. Lesnik, Milton J., and Anderson, Bernice E.: *Nursing Practice and the Law,* 2d ed. Philadelphia, J. B. Lippincott, 1962, p. 261 ff.
63. Woodlawn Infirmary v. Byers, 216 Ala. 210, 112 So. 831 (1927)
64. Criss v. Angelus Hospital Assn., 13 Cal. App. 2d 412, 56 P. 2d 1274 (1936)
65. Inderbitzen *et al.* v. Lane Hospital, 124 Cal. App. 462, 7 P. 2d 1049, 12 P. 2d 744, 13 P. 2d 905 (1932), 61 P. 2d 514 (1936)
66. Taaje v. St. Olaf's Hospital, 271 N.W. 109 (Minn., 1937)
67. Robey v. Jewish Hospital of Brooklyn, 280 N.Y. 533, 21 N.E. 694, 254 App. Div. 874, 5 N.Y.S. 2d 14, 20 N.E. 2d 6 (1939)
68. Pink v. Slater, 131 Cal. App. 2d 816, 13 Am. L. Rep. 2d 11, 281 P. 2d 272 (1955)
69. Thompson v. Methodist Hospital, 211 Tn. 650, 367 S.W. 2d 134 (1963)
70. Helman v. Sacred Heart Hospital, 62 Wash. Rep. 2d 69, 381 P. 2d 605 (1963)
71. Prosser, William L.: *Handbook of Law of Torts,* Sec. 43, St. Paul, West Pub. Co., 1941
72. Valentine v. Kaiser Foundation Hospital, 15 Cal. Rep. 26 (1961)
73. Moore v. Belt, 34 Cal. 2d 525, 203 P. 2d 22, 212 P. 2d 509 (1949)
74. Wallstedt v. Swedish Hospital, 220 Minn. 274, 19 N.W. 2d 426 (1945)
75. Kapuschinsky v. United States, 248 F. Supp. 732 (U.S. D.C. South Carolina, 1966)
76. Beale: The Proximate Consequences of an Act. 33 *Harvard Law Review,* 637 (1920)
77. Valentin v. La Société Française de Bienfaisance Mutuelle de Los Angeles, 76 Cal. App. 2d 1, 172, P. 2d 359 (1956)
78. Chalmers-Francis v. Nelson, 6 Cal. 2d 402, 57 P. 2d 1312 (1936); *Hospitals,* X, 107 (Sept., 1936)
79. Hallinan v. Prindle, 220 Cal. 46, 11 P. 2d 426 (Modified); 17 Cal. App. 2d 656, (Rev'd), 62 P. 2d 1075 Aff'm in Part, (Rev'd in Part 1936). See Gordon, Turner and Price: *Medical Jurisprudence* (1953), p. 148, for an interesting comment and comparison with English cases.
80. Covington v. Wyatt, 196 N.C. 367, 145 S.E. 673 (1928)
81. Iterman v. Baker, 214 Ind. 308, 11 N.E. 2d 64 (1937)
82. Criss v. Angelus Hospital Association of Los Angeles *et al.,* 13 Cal. App. 2d 412, 56 P. 2d 1274 (1936)
83. 128 Mass. 131 (1880)
84. Price v. Neyland, 320 F. 2d 674 (U.S. Ct. of Appeals, Dist. of Columbia, 1963)
85. 235 N.E. 2d 793 (Mass., 1968)
86. James, Charles, Jr.: Lawsuits Involving Nurses Show Need for Individual Coverage. *Hosp. Topics,* 45: 31, July, 1967
87. *Idem.*
88. Kostka, Steve L.: Administrator Has Important Role in Preventing, Fighting Malpractice Suits. *Hosp. Topics,* 46:24, July, 1968
89. Heinz, C. H.: Professional Liability Insurance for Nurses. *Nurs. Clin. of N. Am.,* 2 (1) 175-180 (Mar., 1967), p. 177
90. City of Miami v. Oates, 152 Fla. 21, 10 So. 2d 721 (1942)

General References

Bund, Emanuel: What Nursing Home Administrators Should Know about Drug Regulations. *Nursing Home Administrator,* 20:6-10, May/June, 1966

Crotin, Gloria G.: Medicolegal Problems Can Arise in the Coronary Care Unit. *Canad. Nurse,* 65:37-39, Apr., 1969

Hershey, Nathan: What Is Legal Duty in Infection Control? *Mod. Hosp.,* 105:87-90, July, 1965

Joint Commission on Accreditation of Hospitals: Bulletin No. 35, Surgical Assistants, Chicago, JCAH, Mar., 1964

Regan, William A.: Hospital Nurses and Equipment Failures. *Regan Report on Nursing Law,* 9 (6) 1, Nov., 1968 Patients and Their Personal Effects. *Regan Report on Nursing Law.* 8 (4) 4, Sept., 1967

Chapter Eight

Torts as a Source of Other Civil Actions

TORT DIFFERENTIATED FROM CRIME

At the outset it may be well to differentiate torts from crimes. A tort is a legal wrong, committed against a person or property independent of contract, which renders the person who commits it liable for damages in a civil action. There are many types of torts, but we are interested in the ones most frequently encountered by nurses. A tort or legal wrong may consist of a direct invasion of some legal right of a person, the violation of some public duty by which special damages come to a person, or the violation of some private duty by which damages come to a person.[1]

According to the law of torts, a person, A, is liable for invading (encroaching upon) the interest of another person, B, if the interest invaded is protected against the unintentional invasion, if the conduct of Person A is negligent in regard to such an interest, if such conduct is a legal cause of the invasion, and if Person B has not disabled himself by his conduct so that he is prevented from bringing an action.[2]

By contrast, a *crime* is defined as any wrong which is punishable by the state. For an act to be a deliberate crime, at least two elements are necessary: evil intent (*mens rea*) and a criminal act. However, there are crimes in which the matter of intent is not spelled out; that is, when there is some grossly negligent act or when the person is ignorant of the law.

EXPLANATION OF A CIVIL ACTION

At this junction it is advisable to set forth a brief account of how a civil action proceeds, without attempting a detailed description. In a civil lawsuit, the plaintiff is sometimes called a petitioner and the defendant the respondent. For the court to acquire jurisdiction (a legal right to hear the case), a summons is served on the defendant. A summons is a written notification, signed by the proper officer, served on a person requesting him to appear in court on a specified day to answer to the plaintiff upon pain of judgment against the defendant for default (failure) in not showing up.[3] Pleadings in the case are the papers stating the claims of the plaintiff and the defenses of the defendant.

Before the defendant may be brought to a civil trial, a complaint setting forth the cause of action in legal form must be served upon him. Sometimes the details of the claim are given in a bill of particulars. Then, in return, the defendant sets forth an answer in which he may deny any or all of the plaintiff's charges and offer certain specific defenses, such as the statute of limitations. Alternatively, the defendant may admit all the plaintiff's charges and file a demurrer, which means that, assuming the truth of the charges stated, they do not state a cause of action and hence the plaintiff should not be allowed to proceed further. The defendant may also set up a counter-claim for damages from the plaintiff. After the pleadings have been made, either the plaintiff or the defendant may serve a notice of trial on the other.

Witnesses are served a subpoena, a summons to attend court under a penalty for failure, such as punishment for contempt. At this point, nurses are reminded that one of the obligations or duties of a citizen is to aid the administration of justice and to appear and testify to their knowledge of facts. When a witness must bring certain records, he is served a subpoena known as a *subpoena duces tecum.* The constitutional right of trial by jury may be waived if both plaintiff and defendant agree to do so; in that event the case is tried only before a judge. The right to a trial by jury does not exist in every type of case, but in this brief overview, to give a nurse some notion of civil actions, exceptions and details are omitted. If the trial is by jury, the jurors are selected and sworn (i.e., they take an oath). The trial judge handles questions of law and some questions of fact. Other matters, such as the amount of damages, the trustworthiness of witnesses, and the important question of choosing between conflicting accounts of the events, are left to the jury to decide.

At a civil trial, the plaintiff's lawyer outlines his case and calls his witnesses. The witnesses are then examined by the plaintiff's lawyer; they may be cross-examined by the defendant's lawyer. After this they may be re-examined by the plaintiff's lawyer. When the plaintiff has finished presenting his case, the defendant's lawyer may ask that the suit be dismissed on the ground that the plaintiff has failed to state a case for the defendant to answer. If this is refused, the defendant's case is presented in the same way as was the plaintiff's case. Then follows argument by the lawyers, a "summing up" to the jury. The court instructs the jury as to the law and possible verdicts, after which the jury leaves the courtroom. The jury, in the jury room, weighs the facts and arguments. The jurors return when they are ready either to give a verdict or to state that they cannot reach an agreement. At times, verdicts of juries are set aside as contrary to the law or evidence. One or both of the parties may appeal the decision of a lower court to a higher court.

ASSAULT AND BATTERY

A recital of civil actions other than negligence or malpractice may now be set forth. Assault and battery are two words we often hear together, but they have separate meanings. Assault is the unjustifiable attempt to touch another person or the threat to do so in such circumstances as to cause the other reasonably to believe that it will be carried out.[4] Battery means the unlawful beating of another or the carrying out of threatened physical harm. It includes every willful, angry and violent or negligent touching of another's person or clothes or anything attached to his person or held by him.[5]

Lack of Consent or Privilege

The lack of consent or privilege is an important part of the meaning of assault. Consent is a defense to an action when a person is charged with intentionally interfering with either a person or his property.[6] However, if a person in his actions goes beyond the limits to which a person consented, he may be liable. Also, if the person who does consent is known to be an infant, mentally incompetent or intoxicated—matters which make a person incapable of giving consent—then the consent is not a valid defense. At times, too, physicians and nurses have learned "the hard way" that the fact that treatment is desirable does not allow one to go ahead without the consent of the patient or someone entitled to give consent for him. However, as explained elsewhere, in an emergency a nurse may do what she can to save life and limb, even in cases in which she has no consent or can obtain none. Consent may be given by conduct as well as by express words. For example, when a person held up his arm to be vaccinated, the court said he would not be heard to deny that he had consented.[7] Consent to an act which is *prima facie* (on the surface of it) actionable will afterward deprive a person of the right to complain of it. Although consent may be given by words or implied by conduct, it must be free, and the person must understand what he is doing.

Nurses are concerned about consent forms, and rightly so. In recent years, more and more lawsuits have alleged lack of consent. To begin with, the nurse should know that the attending surgeon has the duty of informing the patient concerning the nature of the proposed surgical procedure.[8] This must be done by a physician and it cannot be delegated to a nurse. Ward secretaries, aides or nurses can fill out the consent form, and any of these people may witness the patient's signing the consent. Preferably, the nurse or physician should present the form to the patient for his signature, since they can more readily appraise his condition at the time. If the patient's sensorium is clouded by medications, such as narcotics, or if he does not know the essential information pertaining to the surgery, he cannot give a valid consent for it. Moreover, the consent must be voluntary, for it is an established principle of the law that an adult of sound mind has the right to decide what shall or shall not be done to his body. In the case of a married woman, her consent is all that is required by law. However, where the surgery affects the sex functions or may result in the death of an unborn child, then as a matter of good public relations the spouse's consent is desirable. Although oral consent, if proved, is valid, written consent is highly desirable and quite generally required by hospitals: Written consents are presumed to be valid, but oral consents may be difficult to prove.

In an emergency, consent may be implied if immediate surgery is necessary to save the patient's life and an express consent cannot be obtained. Consent never authorizes unnecessary surgery.

If the patient is a minor, or at least not a mature or emancipated minor, consent for surgery must be obtained from the parent or guardian. In the case of children whose parents are separated or divorced, consent must be obtained from the parent who has custody. For years, in most states, the physician was liable to charges of assault and battery if he treated the minor without the parents' consent, except in an emergency. In accident cases, such as one in which amputation was necessary to save a 15-year-old boy whose foot was mangled,[9] or one in which a 7-year-old sustained a comminuted fracture of the elbow,[10] the law implied a consent. Also, in a case in which a school principal failed to locate the mother and took a 7-year-old child with a fractured forearm to a doctor's office for treatment, the court held that the physician was justified in proceeding without the parents' consent.[11]

However, when a visiting nurse took a 9-year-old boy to the city doctor, who sent him to a hospital with the request that his tonsils and adenoids be removed, and no one secured the permission of the parents for surgery, the court allowed nominal damages in a suit against the surgeon.[12] Although the boy was accompanied by a 15-year-old brother, such a sibling cannot give a valid consent in lieu of the parents, and this was not an emergency situation.

In the case of a mature minor, his consent may be sufficient, as it was when a 19-year-old boy had a tumor removed from his ear.[13] More recently, in the case of an 18-year-old who had plastic surgery performed on her nose without the consent of her parents, the court held that an unemancipated minor may consent to a "simple operation."[14] However, the parents' responsibility for a child's health and welfare is supported by law, and most physicians and many agencies are reluctant to interfere.

The whole issue of parents' constitutional rights versus a child's right of protection was reviewed in a recent Wisconsin case in which the mother of a 6-year-old Negro boy with sickle-cell anemia refused to give her consent for a splenectomy and other blood procedures recommended by attending physicians, and the State Child Welfare Division filed a petition alleging neglect in failing to provide care necessary for her child's health. The mother objected as a Jehovah's Witness on religious grounds and also:

> . . . because of risks of adverse effects and because medical opinion could not assure her with any certainty that such transfusions would save the life of her child or substantially benefit his health and welfare.[15]

Although the religious objections were overruled, the court found that the mother's:

> . . . reservations and objections to the proposed treatments were made in good faith, entirely apart from her objections for religious reasons.[16]

They dismissed the petition against her.

However, a new Maryland law[17] makes provision for physicians to examine and treat minors for venereal disease without consent of their parents or guardians. Both Massachusetts and Connecticut have somewhat similar statutes.[18] Since many physicians report that minors seek medical prescriptions for "the pill" to prevent conception or for treatment of an illegitimate pregnancy, these statutes are significant, and both nurses and physicians will be obliged to keep their knowledge current in this area.

In one case, the Supreme Court of Illinois held that the appointment of a conservator and authorization of transfusions of whole blood to a ward without giving notice to her or to her husband interfered with their basic constitutional rights. The couple had notified the physician and hospital of their belief that the acceptance of blood transfusions constituted a violation of the law of God, no minor children were involved, and there appeared otherwise no clear and present danger to society.[19]

When an operating room supervisor is or ought to be aware of the performance of an unusual surgical procedure, she is responsible for notifying her nursing supervisor if the consent for surgery lacks reference to such a procedure.[20] When a minor died following a very unusual surgical procedure for scoliosis, and the surgeon had not informed the parents of the unusual procedure, but the hospital knew he had used it for several years, both the surgeon and the hospital were liable in damages.[21] The nurse who finds herself unexpectedly assisting a surgeon who is doing something unusual or something that is even in violation of hospital rules must continue to assist the surgeon, for to do otherwise might jeopardize the patient's life. However, after surgery she should report the matter to her superior in the chain of command.

It is sometimes difficult for a nurse to realize that a person does not have to accept treatment and be healed, and that treatment must not be forced upon him. In discussing consents, Grace Barbee, lawyer for the California Nurses' Association, cites a Long Island case in which the physician thought a patient who had been seriously ill should be motivated to get out of bed and walk. All efforts to motivate him failed, so the physician threw back the bed covers and he and the nurse slid the patient to the floor and carefully walked him around and then put him back to bed. Some days later, the patient was discharged. However, the patient sued the physician and hospital for damages for assault and battery, and the court allowed the suit on the grounds that the patient had an absolute right to refuse to be touched.[22]

Research Consents

If nurses are not to share the headlines with other clinical investigators,[23] they must secure the patient's consent in research. Any research should provide that the subject patient will be given sufficient information so that he can make a knowledgeable decision as to whether he wishes to participate in the study. The abuses in drug evaluation studies prompted the Food and Drug Administration to issue specific guidelines on how patient consent is to be obtained. The new guidelines state:

> The patient must have the legal capacity and freedom of choice to give consent, and . . . he must be given necessary information about the investigational drug. This information must include the purpose of the drug, the duration and method of use, hazards expected (including the fact that the patient may be used

as a control), alternative therapy available, if any, and possible effects upon his health.[24]

The guidelines say that the "not feasible" exemption will be:

> . . . limited to cases where the patient cannot communicate or is otherwise unable to give his informed consent, his representative is not available, and it is necessary to use the drug without delay.

A patient brought a million-dollar suit against the Memorial Hospital for Cancer and Allied Diseases, the Memorial Sloan-Kettering Cancer Center, the Sloan-Kettering Institute for Cancer Research, and the James Ewing Hospital, a city institution, charging that he was injected with live cancer cells. The patient had been suffering from cancer for some years. The experiments were part of a 10-year study by the Sloan-Kettering Center designed to test the speed and manner in which debilitated noncancerous patients reject cancer implants.[25]

Examples of Assault and Battery

Freedom from contact with another person is one of our personal rights, and this applies to the nurse-patient relationship. When a person comes to the hospital, presumably he consents to be treated, and at times this involves contact with another person. However, he may have some ideas of his own, and he may wish to refuse certain contacts, and may say so. For example, he may refuse a back rub or an intramuscular injection of a drug. In such a case, if the nurse, for instance, knowing that a paralyzed patient has refused to consent to such an injection, nevertheless comes toward him with 2 cc. of penicillin in a syringe with a No. 22 needle in her hand as though she were going to give him an injection, she has threatened or assaulted him even though she says nothing. If she follows through, still without his consent, and gives him the injection, the nurse has committed a battery.

A nurse may be liable on a charge of battery if she does anything improper in handling or treating an unconscious patient. One does not need to be in actual person-to-person contact to commit a battery. If a person strikes another with a stick or rolled paper, or forcibly removes clothing without the other's consent, it may be an act of battery.

On the other hand, it may be that the nurse has to defend herself against the patient, who might assault or strike her. This might happen, for instance, in psychiatric nursing. Everyone is allowed to defend himself from unlawful attack. However, only those steps necessary for self-protection or the aid of another are permitted. Self-defense is said to extend to the use of reasonable force which appears to be necessary for protection against the threatened interference.[26] A few cases illustrating action involving assault are given.

In a Pennsylvania case, an agent of an artificial limb company falsely represented himself as a physician to a woman who had lost one leg and wore an artificial one, and she was persuaded therefore to undress so that he could determine how it fitted. Under these circumstances, the fraud negated her consent, and the man was held guilty of indecent assault.[27] Most actions involving assault and battery are brought as civil actions to recover damages, but this example illustrates how they may be criminal proceedings, with the state prosecuting a person for his act.

In a New York case, in which the parents of an 11-year-old boy sued physicians to recover damages for the boy's death, on the grounds that they had performed an unnecessary operation without the consent of the patient, of his parents or of a person in whose custody the boy was, the doctor offered evidence that the boy had blood poisoning, that he acted in an emergency, and that the use of chloroform as an anesthetic was reasonable, although it proved fatal to the boy because of status lymphaticus. The judgment was for the physicians.[28]

In a Louisiana case, the defendant was infuriated one morning by the way the plaintiff drove his car, and he followed him to a parking lot in the city. A fight followed, during which the plaintiff had his clothes torn and his face bruised. An award of $350 caused by unprovoked assault and battery was held not excessive in view of the plaintiff's injuries, embarrassment and humiliation, in addition to damage to his clothing. The court observed:

> No provocative acts, conduct, former insults, threats, or words, if unaccompanied by any overt act of hostility, will justify an assault, no matter how offensive or exasperating, nor how much they can be calculated to excite or irritate.[29]

An Iowa case concerned an action for damages for assault and battery wherein the plaintiff offered evidence that the defendant maliciously assaulted him, causing severe pain, injury and humiliation and requiring medical treatment, and disabled him from attending his business for five days. A verdict for $500 for actual damages and $500 exemplary damages was upheld.[30]

In a Tennessee case, a corporation and doctors employed by the corporation in a dispensary for treating employees were not liable for damages when the plaintiff charged that her examination by the physicians, since they lacked a state license to practice medicine, was really assault and battery, even though she had voluntarily submitted to the examination on the supposition that the physicians were licensed. The plaintiff did not claim any negligent acts on the part of the physicians in their diagnosis or treatment, nor did she claim that the corporation was negligent in selecting the doctors. The court said that failure to comply with a licensing statute might subject a person to criminal prosecution. Nevertheless, to sustain a civil action on these facts, the plaintiff must show that the result complained of was due to negligent or unskilled treatment.[31]

A person is allowed to defend another person by use of force reasonably necessary to prevent a threatened attack when the defense would be allowed by ordinary social custom.[32] Also, one who has real or personal property is allowed to defend it by the use of force which appears reasonably necessary to prevent threatened interference with his possession.[33]

As one writer has pointed out in discussing torts, it is justifiable to violate a police regulation in order to save a life.[34] As a parent may use reasonable force in the correction and punishment of a child, so may military officers use similar disciplinary authority. In some jurisdictions, a school teacher also may use disciplinary measures involving reasonable force or restraint to maintain morale and order. Likewise, a person may, if necessary, use reasonable force in resisting an unlawful arrest.

In discussing intent in tort actions, a well-known authority has said that a person intends a result when he acts in order to achieve it or when the result is certain to follow from his acts.[35]

Persons acting unlawfully, or not conducting themselves properly, may be ejected forcibly from a building if necessary. This could happen to a nurse if she were incompetent or her conduct were unprofessional, e.g., if she were inebriated when she came on duty. If, when requested by the hospital to leave, she did not go quietly, she could be ejected forcibly.

When a private duty registered nurse was injured by an alcoholic patient who hit her on the head with a table lamp, she sued him for assault.[36] The state supreme court reversed a verdict for the patient and ordered a new trial, stating that she assumed the risk of injury if she could have prevented it by the exercise of due care or if it was not an unreasonable risk for her to accept in the course of her duty. A private duty nurse is an independent contractor. Consent is a defense to assault and battery cases as well as others, unless the consent is against the policy of the law. The defense of assumption of risk comes from the common law rule of *volenti non fit injuria;* i.e., to one who consents no wrong is done.

In an action by a patient against a sanitarium for injuries including a fractured jaw when he was struck by an employee upon the chin, an adverse judgment was affirmed because it appeared that the attendant committed assault and battery in his own necessary self-defense.[37]

A patient who sustained a fractured jaw when assaulted and beaten by an attendant who objected to his tapping his foot on the floor at the Brooklyn State Hospital, to which he was confined, recovered $3000 damages for pain and suffering.[38] The court stated that the state must exercise reasonable care to protect its patients from injuries with such attention to their safety and the safety of others as their mental and physical condition, if known, may require. New York is one of the few states that does permit patients in its state hospitals to bring suit against the state.

Nurses have been concerned about whether they could draw a blood sample when requested by the police in the absence of the patient's consent. In *Schmerber v. State of California,* the Supreme Court of the United States ruled that the tests made on a blood sample drawn by a physician in a hospital from a person arrested by the police were admissible evidence in a court action.[39] Nurses should check on the state law in the state in which they are working, as such laws vary. Whereas Kansas rules that a blood sample is not to be withdrawn if the person objects, although such refusal is a basis for suspending his driver's license,[40] New York exempts physicians, registered professional nurses and their employers from liability if they draw a blood sample without the person's consent at the request of the police.[41]

CHILD ABUSE

Not all parents are reasonable and prudent, let alone loving; some few frankly abuse their children in fits of anger or for various other reasons. Therefore, all states in recent years have enacted laws to encourage or compel people to report any suspected case of child abuse to the police or child welfare agency and provide immunity from civil and criminal suit for those who do. In the following states, nurses must report child abuse: New York, Pennsylvania, Maryland, Virginia, West Virginia, North Carolina, South Carolina, Georgia, Alabama, Mississippi, Tennessee, Kentucky, Ohio, Wisconsin, North Dakota, Minnesota, Iowa, Kansas, Nebraska, Utah, Wyoming, Montana, Nevada, New Mexico, Arkansas, Oklahoma, Alaska and Hawaii.[42] About half the states require only doctors and/or other personnel to report child abuse, whereas a few states require everyone to report it. Along with the reporting required by law, the nurse who is knowledgeable in the services of community agencies may often refer these people to those equipped to help them deal with their problems.

Statutes give juvenile courts jurisdiction over "neglected" children in every state, and mistreatment is a form of neglect. In some states, the emphasis is on the behavior of the parent, for example, whether he is cruel to a child. In other states, the emphasis is on the child's environment and whether it is unsuitable, due to the neglect of a parent or parents. What the statute of a particular state emphasizes is important, since it tells what must be proven to spell out a neglect case. In any neglect or child abuse case, two questions have to be answered: (1) what actually happened and (2) do the facts presented amount to neglect or abuse?

Evidence is a problem, and situations about which objective proof cannot be produced cannot be remedied through the court. However, at least in one state, circumstantial evidence may shift the burden of a satisfactory explanation to the parents. For instance, In the Matter of S., the court said:

> . . . the proceeding . . . was initiated undoubtedly by a consensus of view, medical and social agency, that the child Freddie, only a month old, presented a case of a battered child syndrome. Proof of abuse by a parent or parents is difficult because such actions ordinarily occur in the privacy of the home without outside witnesses. Objective study of the problem of the battered child . . . has pointed up a number of propositions, among them, that usually it is only one child in the family who is the victim; that the parents tend to protect each other and resist outside inquiry and interference; and that the adult who has injured a child tends to repeat such action and suffers no remorse from his conduct.
>
> Therefore in this type of proceedings affecting a battered child syndrome, I am borrowing from the evidentiary law of negligency the principle of "res ipsa loquitor" and accepting the proposition that the condition of the child speaks for itself, thus permitting an inference of neglect to be drawn from proof of the child's age and condition, and that the latter is such as in the ordinary course of things does not happen if the parent who has the responsibility and control of the infant is protective and nonabusive. And without satisfactory explanation, I would be constrained to make a finding of fact of neglect on the part of the parent or parents and thus afford the court the opportunity to inquire into any mental, physical or emotional inadequacies of the parents and/or to enlist any guidance and counseling the parents might need. This is the Court's responsibility to the Child.[43]

In such situations, the juvenile court may order protective supervision of the child so that his situation may be improved through casework techniques and the use of other community resources. In some states, the welfare department is required to investigate and offer social services to families where child abuse is alleged.[44]

As Cheney has pointed out,[45] the problem of safeguarding legal rights in providing protective services is a thorny one. In those states which have no statutes for providing protective services in child neglect cases, then under juvenile court laws, the parent is protected from state power by the requirements of due process of law. However, in protective services, the social worker who is part of an administrative agency is authorized to supervise the home as the court may order, and the standards of care expected of the family are set by the agency at its discretion. The presence of a stranger (the agency worker) in the home may deprive parents of liberty without due process of law. In addition, the due process requirement raises the family's right to counsel at a hearing. Because juvenile court hearings do not have to provide a defendant with the same safeguards as are necessarily provided in a criminal action, providing the family with counsel in the form of a lawyer is not mandatory. As a consequence, many feel the legal maxim that "every man is entitled to his day in court" is not carried into effect and that administrative agencies with supposedly benevolent intentions negate legal rights in a number of instances.

That the actions of the protective services are not without question or criticism by various members of society is illustrated by some of the following cases: A complaint of neglect was brought because the child's parents advocated Communism,[46] because their interracial marriage affected the family-community relationship,[47] and because they neglected the child's religious instruction.[48] While one family was petitioning for a reversal of a decision denying them the return of their children because their house was too small, they lost half of them through adoption.[49] Also, one agency petitioned to remove a child from his home because his mother visited taverns.[50] Therefore, as Cheney points out, the best way to assure both that due process of law is followed and that the values on which decisions are made are clearly stated is to provide parents with counsel.[51] Legal procedures are not impediments to timely correction of this social ill of child abuse, but they would help to make certain that the decisions of protective services are based on relevant criteria.

School nurses should protect themselves from possible lawsuits by making certain that their reports are made only to designated individuals within the school system. Since the school nurse and social welfare people are often among the first people to know of child abuse, the school nurse's reports on this matter are important.[52]

Foster parents were convicted of manslaughter in the death of a 4-year-old child who died from a hematoma caused by a subdural hemorrhage and aggravated by a second skull injury. The child's body showed marks of over 150 bruises of varying ages. The parents stated that the child was extremely clumsy and sustained the injuries in two falls down the stairs.[53]

FALSE IMPRISONMENT

False imprisonment means the unjustifiable detention of a person without a legal warrant within boundaries fixed by the defendant by an act or violation of duty intended to result in such confinement.[54] For example, to confine a patient by locking him in a room unjustifiably is a false imprisonment. If it is accompanied by unjustifiable forcible restraint or threat of restraint, it is an assault. In regard to nurses and other medical personnel, the charge of false imprisonment may arise in the case of mental patients. To prevent injury to himself or others or to prevent property damage, a right existed at common law to confine an insane person. However, this right existed only for the length of time required to get legal authority for the person's restraint. By statutes in the various states today, procedures have been devised for committing persons who are mentally deranged and for caring for their property.

Another way in which a charge of false imprisonment may arise against a nurse might be for detaining a patient for payment of a bill. A nurse, for example, may detain a patient for a few minutes to check on whether he has paid his bill, and this is looked upon as reasonable and permissible. She may not, however, lawfully detain such a patient longer, whether he has or has not paid the bill. The detention of a patient for failure to pay his bill would be false imprisonment. There are other remedies available to a person at law for collecting wages, payment for services and hospital charges.

For example, a sane person was kept for 11 hours in a hospital against her will for failure to pay a bill. There was evidence that one of the nurses told her she would be tied to the bed if she did not keep quiet. and that the door was locked. The plaintiff recovered money damages.[55]

In another case, a dentist in his office claimed that a patient owed him $33 for denture work. The patient asserted that the fees amounted to $22; the dentist locked the door to compel her to pay what he claimed or return the denture. The patient sued him for damages for false imprisonment, and the dentist was adjudged liable.[56]

A suit against a hospital for false imprisonment of a child was dismissed in a case in which the mother, who had come to take her child home from the hospital, was delayed 30 minutes while she arranged for payment of her child's bill.[57] Since there was no threat that unless the bill was paid or secured the child could not leave the hospital, the charge of false imprisonment was not supported.

A patient discharged from Mattewan State Hospital was awarded $300,000 in damages for false imprisonment.[58] The facts of the case show he had been committed to this hospital for the criminally insane with a diagnosis of a paranoid condition with chronic alcoholism in May, 1947, when he was incompetent to stand criminal trial for assault with a knife. At the trial, various psychiatric witnesses testified that with proper treatment he should be discharged within two years at the most and sent back for trial. Accordingly, he was given damages for the balance of his 12 years and four months of confinement. The case stands for the right to treatment. If this case is followed, then a patient can sue for a writ of *habeas corpus* and compel his release from a psychiatric hospital on the grounds of no or inadequate treatment.

Saralee Maniaci, a former student, sued Marquette University for false imprisonment and libel and a physician for malpractice and asked $300,000 damages from each for being placed in a hospital mental ward when she tried to quit college without saying where she was going. As a 16-year-old boarding student living far from her parents, she was blocked by university officials who first wanted to contact her parents. The doctor said she told him that she was going to work in a nightclub and support herself. She was released the next morning when her father called and demanded she be freed.[59]

ALCOHOLICS AND PUBLIC DRUNKENNESS

Those nurses who work with alcoholics will be interested in the *Powell v. State of Texas* decision. Although the court recognized alcoholism as one of the most serious social and public health problems in current society, it described professional knowledge of the subject as "comparatively primitive." Consequently, the court refused to rule that the criminal punishment of a chronic alcoholic for public drunkenness was unconstitutional. Said the court:

> One virtue of the criminal process is, at least, that the duration of penal incarceration typically has some outside statutory limit . . . therapeutic civil commitment lacks this feature; one is typically committed until one is "cured." Thus, to do otherwise than affirm [the conviction of Powell], might subject indigent alcoholics to the risk that they may be locked up for an indefinite period of time under the same conditions as before, with no more hope than before of receiving effective treatment and no prospect of periodic "freedom."[60]

To convict an ambulance driver of driving while under the influence of liquor, some courts require chemical evidence and others merely use common sense.[61]

RESTRAINT OF FREEDOM OF MOVEMENT

Restraint of freedom of movement of a patient by a nurse is at times a problem involving such factors as safety, negligence, and false imprisonment. Restraining a patient's movements is sometimes necessary, but care, caution and reasonableness in so doing for the patient's safety and welfare must be used. The use of side rails on beds of postoperative patients under the influence of anesthesia or the elderly patient at night, of crib sides on the beds of children, and rarely, on a doctor's order, of other mechanical restraints on irrational or violent patients, is a common procedure when properly applied in hospitals. With the advent of the modern tranquilizing drugs and their use in institutions for the mentally ill, the recourse to use of mechanical restraints and of seclusion rooms will be further lessened.

INVASION OF PRIVACY

Invasion of a person's privacy may constitute a legal wrong. Actions are sometimes brought for damages for invading a person's right of privacy.[62] A nurse, particularly in the case of patients with unusual conditions or operations, can appreciate how photographers or writers (medical and otherwise) might be tempted to invade this right or extend a limited consent. At times, some patients simply dislike even the least unnecessary scrutiny. Understandably, caution must be taken against a violation of their right of privacy. The right of privacy is the right of an individual to withhold himself and his property from public scrutiny.[63] No person can enjoy complete isolation, but rather, as a citizen in our democratic society, has duties which require disclosures in the public interest. However, a tort action may be brought against a person who seriously or unreasonably interferes with another's privacy by having his affairs made known or his likeness exhibited in public.[64]

For example, in a Georgia case, the parents of a deceased child brought a petition against a hospital, photographer and newspaper for damages and to enjoin the unauthorized publication of a picture of their son, who was born with his heart on the outside of his body. He had been taken to the hospital, and the operation could not correct the defect, which resulted in death. The parents alleged that the privacy of their lives had been invaded, inflicting much anguish and mental suffering. A judgment for the defendant was reversed on appeal.[65]

In a Michigan case in which a doctor allowed an unmarried nonprofessional man in the delivery room, the plaintiff recovered substantial damages for her injured feelings.[66] There has been much criticism of this case, but it does impress upon a nurse, to whom deliveries, operations, examinations and treatments appear routine, the need to consider the right of privacy and how her public regards that right.

Another case which may be of interest concerned a woman who had been a prostitute and was acquitted of murder. After the trial, she abandoned her life of shame, became rehabilitated, married and lived an exemplary life for seven years before the moving picture was made. She had assumed a place in respectable society, and acquired friends not aware of incidents in her earlier years. The plaintiff was held entitled to recover damages from the producer of "The Red Kimono," which was a film based on the true story of her past life and used the plaintiff's true maiden name. All the facts of the script were in records available to the public eye. In this case, the court was hesitant to recognize the right of privacy as a basis of an action for tort in the absence of a statute. Nevertheless, the court based its decision on the provision of the state constitution, conferring upon citizens the right of:

... procuring and obtaining safety and happiness.[67]

A patient has every right to keep himself from unnecessary and unauthorized public exposure or scrutiny. This means that the publication of his picture in a magazine or newspaper or other periodical without his consent may be a tort constituting an invasion of the right of privacy. The person who is guilty of permitting the invasion is answerable at law. A nurse should guard against such intrusion. However, there is no tort when the person is a public figure or does acts of public interest.

DEFAMATION

Defamation is another wrongful action. A nurse should be careful in her personal statements, especially regarding patients, doctors, hospital supervisors and fellow workers. Unquestionably, one way that nurses sometimes get into trouble is by making unguarded derogatory remarks. Granted, legal actions arising therefrom are the exception; nevertheless, the volume of criticism of such conduct is appreciable. As a student, each nurse has been taught that it is wrong to discuss patients except in so far as their care necessitates such discussion in a professional setting.

An invasion of a person's interest in his reputation and good name by communication to others of anything which tends to diminish the value or esteem in which he is held or to arouse adverse feelings against him is defamation.[68] Defamation consists of publication of matter which tends to lower the reputation of a person or to cause ordinary reasonable persons to shun him. A nurse may defame a patient, or a patient may defame a nurse. Not every mentioning of a person's affairs is defamatory, but only such things as engender derogatory opinions of others. For example, to say that a patient had a common cold or fractured arm could hardly be considered defamatory. On the other hand, to say that a patient had a venereal disease would be defamatory. Likewise, to say that a patient had a mental disease or some unpleasant physical deformity might be considered defamatory. In many jurisdictions, to publish that an unmarried woman is pregnant is defamatory, since it carries a charge of immoral behavior.[69] It is also defamatory to cast any reflection on a person's fitness or ability for his work.

Slander and Libel

Under the title of defamation, the law in many states draws a distinction between slander and libel. Slander is the oral defamation of a person by speaking unprivileged or false words by which his reputation is damaged.[70] Libel is printed defamation by written words, cartoons, effigies, and such representations as cause a person to be avoided, ridiculed or held in contempt, or tend to injure him in his work.[71]

Neither of these two types of defamation of character applies to remarks between two persons that are directed at each other. There must be a third person to hear or read the comment before it can be considered "published." For instance, a nurse might make a contemptuous remark about a patient, physician or another nurse to the person himself. This would not constitute slander. But if the contemptuous remark was made in the presence of a third person, it would be slander. Or, if the nurse made a remark of this type to another nurse or other person about a third person, it would constitute slander.

Similarly, a statement is not libel even if it is written to another, provided it is not seen by a third person. It is considered "publication" in various jurisdictions if a person has dictated to his secretary the statement complained of in the letter. A nurse should realize, too, that some kinds of defamation are actionable without proof of damage. For instance, a statement that affects a person in his profession or business or says that he is connected with a serious crime would be slander.[72] Some slanderous words — for instance, those imputing lack of chastity to a woman — are by special laws made criminal in some jurisdictions.

A nurse recovered $5000 damages in a slander action against a doctor on the staff of the Cary Memorial Hospital in Caribou, Maine. A feud raged between the doctor and the nurse after the nurse was dismissed by the hospital for unprofessional conduct when she became openly critical of the postoperative treatment being given a patient by the doctor. The charges she brought against the doctor were dismissed by the Grievance Committee of the Aroostook County Medical Association. Some time later she was re-employed by the hospital upon the stated condition that she not discuss hospital business outside the hospital. When the physician learned that the nurse had been re-employed, he called the administrator and said:

> I wanted to ask you if you would stoop so low as to hire that creep, that malignant son of a bitch, back to work for you in the hospital.

He added:

> She was unfit for the care of patients . . . he could prove that . . . and that he intended to make an issue of it.

The nurse learned of these remarks and brought suit against the doctor. If actual malice is shown, the plaintiff may recover compensatory damages and punitive damages. A jury verdict of $17,500 was reduced to $5000 since provocation, although no excuse for slander, is a mitigating factor in assessing punitive damages.[73]

Excuse of Defamatory Statement

The greater the publicity given to a defamatory statement, the greater the damage to the plaintiff's reputation. A defamatory statement may be excused or justified by showing that the person who made it was not moved to do it by a spirit of injury, but for a nonmalicious, justifiable purpose: for example, proof of consent, truth, privilege or fair comment.

There are circumstances when a legal or moral duty exists for a person to pass on information of a defamatory nature to another. A nurse may feel obliged to give a confidential report to a person entitled to it. For example, a director of nursing service in a hospital who has personal knowledge of the character and qualifications of a nurse, Miss Jones, may give her fair opinion of Miss Jones to an employer who is considering hiring her. It is not difficult to decide when there is a legal duty to speak. The nurse must do so when required to give evidence in court and when it is reasonably necessary for the patient's own sake, as in the case of a patient with a deranged mind. But to decide when a person has a moral or social duty to speak is considerably more difficult. Perhaps the only guide in such situations is to ask whether an ordinary, reasonable person under the circumstances would feel obliged to speak.

Again, a person may make a statement to protect her reasonable interest, as in self-defense. An assistant director of nursing service may complain to the director of nursing service about the work of a certain practical nurse on duty in the hospital, but she would not be justified in complaining about irrelevant matters.

Truth. In our law, in the absence of a privileged communication, truth is a good defense in a civil suit for libel or slander. But a nurse should remember that if she resorts to truth as a defense, she must prove the whole defamatory statement to be true and not merely a part of it. Also, if a person relies on the defense of truth and fails to prove it, it would seem that the action has increased the amount of damages which the plaintiff might sue for, since it shows persistence in the defamation and probably gives it wider publicity.

It would seem pertinent at this point to remind nurses of the wisdom of thinking before they speak. Many former student nurses will recall two of my favorite quotations, one attributed to the late President Calvin Coolidge:

> I notice that what I have not said, never gets me into any trouble.

The second is attributed to Halleck and Franz, authors some years ago of a grade-school text on American history:

> The sphinx of Egypt looks wise enough to solve any question and has maintained its reputation through the centuries by saying nothing.

To be sure, there is at times a duty to speak, and then one should.

Many times it has been remarked that there are more needless actions brought for defamation than for any other cause. Before a person initiates suit, she should consider whether it is honestly worth the trouble, time and expense involved. However, if a defamation is particularly damaging, in order to clear her good name, she may be impelled to bring an action against a person even if he is a known pauper from whom recovery would be extremely unlikely.

Under the common law, truth is not a defense to a criminal libel action. In criminal actions, if the publication of the statement is for a justifiable and not a malicious purpose, truth is an available defense.

Privilege. In discussing "privilege," an authority on torts has said that a person may be privileged to publish defamation for protection or furtherance of public or private interests recognized by law.[74] He observed that in one group of actions, such as legal and legislative proceedings, publications made with the consent of the plaintiff, communications between husband and wife, and circumstances in which executive officers are charged with important responsibilities, there is an immunity from responsibility without regard to the defendant's motive or reasonableness. In another set of situations, however, there is a limited or conditional privilege, and there the defendant's immunity depends on good motives and reasonable behavior. Here, by way of illustration, the author cites communications between those having a common interest for the advancement of that interest, publication made to proper persons in the public interest, publications to protect or advance an important interest of the person or a third person in such circumstances as an ordinary reasonable person would consider himself under a moral or legal obligation to do so, and in accounts of proceedings of public interest.[75]

Before concluding this section on wrongs against persons, privileged communications should be discussed further. There are certain classes of confidential or privileged communications between persons who stand in a confidential or fiduciary (founded on or holding in trust) relationship to each other, and for the sake of public policy and the good of society the law will not permit them to be divulged or allow them to be inquired into in a court of justice.[76] Examples of such communications are those between husband and wife, attorney and client, and a clergyman and person who seeks him for counsel.

The common law does not recognize the relationship of physician-patient as confidential or privileged. Privilege between physician and patient is based on the idea that the physician cannot give adequate care to a patient without the patient's completely disclosing the facts relating to his ailment. In about two-thirds of the states, there are statutes providing for privileged communications between physician and patient. Generally, these statutes confer a qualified type of privilege.

States conferring a physician-patient privilege include New York, Ohio, Indiana, Illinois, Michigan, Wisconsin, Minnesota, North Dakota, South Dakota, Iowa, Missouri, Kansas, Nebraska, Oklahoma, Arkansas, Mississippi, Colorado, Wyoming, Utah, Montana, Idaho, Washington, Oregon, California, Arizona, Alaska and Hawaii. The District of Columbia also allows the physician-patient privilege.

Recently, New Jersey enacted a law to protect the confidentiality of communications between a physician and patient.[77] Massachusetts has also enacted a statute to protect the confidential communications between patients and psychotherapists.[78]

In a recent case, an accident victim was in the hospital, and her physician requested Dr. Murtagh, a neurosurgeon, to examine her. When he did examine her, Dr. Murtagh decided that she had sustained a moderately severe whiplash injury to the neck and spine, had marked spasm in the muscles, and that there was a marked hysterical element present which was more severe since the patient was basically emotionally unstable. Dr. Erickson, employed by the defense attorneys to interview doctors of injured patients and secure a report for them, secured a report from Dr. Murtagh without the patient's permission to give such information. In his report, for which he was paid $50 by the doctor for the defense attorneys, Dr. Murtagh stated:

> It is my opinion that there was a very mild musculo-ligamentous strain at the time of the accident but no neurogenic involvement, nothing to suggest a permanent neurologic sequelae, and that the prognosis for recovery of this mild strain should be very good. Her somatic symptoms, however, have been perpetuated by an underlying pre-existing anxiety neurosis and hysteria, centered about an hysterical personality.

Affirming a motion for a new trial because of the verdict inadequacy, the court scored the physicians on privileged communications, saying:

> We are of the opinion that members of a profession, especially the medical profession, stand in a confidential or fiduciary capacity as to their patients. They owe their patients more than just medical care for which payment is exacted; there is a duty of total care; that includes and comprehends a duty to aid the patient in litigation, to render reports when necessary and to attend court when needed.

It also said:

> The doctor, of course, owes a duty to conscience to speak the truth; he need, however, speak only at the proper time. Dr. Erickson's role in inducing Dr. Murtagh's breach of his confidential relationship to his patient is to be and is condemned.[79]

In Louisiana, no physician-patient privilege exists, according to the appellate court. A husband who was legally separated from his wife sued for custody of the two minor children, alleging that the mother was in a psychiatric hospital and unable to care for them. The mother claimed privilege of the information between physician and patient. The court ruled that the issue could not be satisfactorily determined without a full disclosure of the findings of the medical expert who had examined and treated the defendant.[80]

In Georgia, the privilege applies only to communications between a patient and a psychiatrist, and in both Virginia and North Carolina disclosure can be ordered when it is needed in administering justice. Privilege is limited to vital statistics in Kentucky, to information which tends to blacken the character of the patient in Pennsylvania and to workmen's compensation claims and loathesome diseases in New Mexico. In West Virginia, privilege is allowed only in the justice court.

As a rule, however, communications to a nurse are not privileged except by statutes in New York, Arkansas and New Mexico, which have changed the common law rule and have expressly included a professional registered nurse in their scope. As a court in Arkansas pointed out in a suit by a physician against the father of the patient to collect for services to a patient, a statute declaring physicians and nurses to be privileged from compulsion as witnesses concerning certain kinds of testimony has no application to the testimony of a nurse as to a conference between the defendant father of the patient and a plaintiff physician as to his agreement to pay the physician for the patient's operation.[81]

Although a nurse is not specifically mentioned in a privileged communications statute, courts have held that a professional nurse assisting a physician is his agent and therefore, when so acting, stands in the same confidential relation to the patient as the physician himself.

According to a Nebraska decision, a professional nurse assisting a physician to whom a confidential communication is made by a patient is the agent of the physician. Accordingly, no doctor or his agent shall be allowed in giving testimony to disclose any confidential communication entrusted to him in his professional capacity and necessary and proper to enable him to carry on his work according to the usual course of practice. In an action against a railroad company by the administrator of a patient who was a brakeman and had been injured and paralyzed, a judgment in a trial in which such persons had given testimony was reversed.[82]

However, when the information is acquired by a professional nurse unconnected with the patient's treatment and diagnosis, the rule does not hold that the nurse is an agent of the physician and as such prohibited from disclosing confidential communications. In an action to set aside and cancel a deed of property valued at $100,000 to a husband, it was alleged that the woman (patient) was mentally incompetent at the time of executing the deed and that the deed was procured through fraud and undue influence. It was further alleged that the deed was never delivered, and that if it was delivered it was not to take effect until after the death of the patient. The nurse's testimony tended to show that the patient (wife) knew what she was doing, intended to act as she did when she executed the deed, and that it was delivered to the husband. A judgment for the defendant husband was affirmed.[83] In this case, the communications of a patient to a nurse were not necessary to enable the physician to prescribe or treat the patient and were not within the privileged communication law.

In regard to the practical nurse, it would seem that, since she is neither "professional" nor "registered," no communication between the patient and her is privileged, and as a consequence she may be called in an action to testify to what she knows. In a case wherein the plaintiff physician recovered a judgment for services to the defendant's wife, the court said that a nurse who is not registered or professional can properly give testimony of conversations between physician and patient as to the patient's condition and its cause.[84]

In some states, there is no law allowing privileged communications between physician and patient, and hence no law cloaking as privileged any communications between patient and nurse. In an action for damages for death of the plaintiff intestate while riding in an automobile which was struck by a train at a crossing, the court noted that under the common law still in force, confidential communications between physician and patient arising from professional relations were not privileged. The section of the civil code making privileged all communications to attorney by a client or to clergyman or priest when made to him in confidence was inapplicable between physician and patient.[85] Also, in a homicide action wherein a husband had fatally shot his wife, resulting in a first degree murder charge, part of the evidence revealed that the wife was pregnant and did not want a child, while the husband did want a child. Communications between physician and patient (wife) as to the pregnancy, during which the wife told the doctor she wanted him to terminate the pregnancy and he had consented, were admissible. Communications between patient and physician were not privileged in Alabama.[86]

Statements Actionable *Per Se*

As has been previously mentioned, in some cases the words of a statement are "actionable *per se*"; that is, the words are actionable in themselves and damages are presumed and need not be proved. Several actions of this type include accusation of unfitness for a trade or profession, immorality, commission of a serious crime, or having venereal disease. If a physician untruthfully accused a nurse to a third person of unskillfulness because a patient was injured by failure to turn him properly, it probably would be sufficient to constitute slander. The court considered it slander when a defendant doctor said of a nurse:

> Many have perished for want of her skill.[87]

In another case, a doctor sued for slander when the defendant in connection with a confinement case said:

> I heard Doc A was drunk that night and wasn't able to go.

The court held that such a statement was prejudicial to the plaintiff in his profession and actionable as slander.[88]

In an action for libel against a hospital and its secretary in his individual capacity, a physician based his complaint on letters dictated by the defendant secretary to his stenographer. One such letter on the hospital letterhead and signed by the defendant read:

> Dear Sir:
> I am calling your attention to the unpaid hospital bill of Julia Sagert, amounting to $301.24.
> As this girl received treatment following a criminal operation for which you were responsible, we hereby request and demand you make immediate payment of this bill. If you fail to do so, we will institute criminal proceedings and use our best efforts to see you are committed to the state penitentiary.
> This is a final notice and your immediate attention is requested.[89]

The plaintiff, alleging that he was seriously injured and had lost gains and profit in his practice, asked for $10,000 damages. The court said that if the expression in the letter "for which you were responsible" referred to the statement "the unpaid hospital bill," found in the first paragraph, and not to the expression "criminal operation," found in the second paragraph immediately preceding the matter in controversy, it could be shown in defense or mitigation of damages. Also, the court said that if the secretary of the board of trustees of the hospital while in the discharge of duties published a libel, the hospital, in addition to the secretary, was liable for such act and that the hospital was not immune from liability because it was a nonprofit charitable organization.

RESTRAINTS

The problem of the use of restraints at times confronts nurses who care for disoriented, irrational and restless patients. Whatever restraint is used should be adequate for the purpose, but the same type may not always be needed. In some situations, besides restraints, continuing observation by some member of the nursing team may be necessary for the safety of the patient. Therefore, the nurse must know when and how to use restraints correctly; depending on the circumstances, there may or may not be a medical order. Even when patients are restrained, many accidents happen; hence it is well to realize that the use of restraints imposes an obligation on the nurse to observe the patient more frequently and carefully.[90]

A recovery room nurse placed restraining boards on the arms of a 6-year-old girl who had had eye surgery, and she struggled against them. When the restraints were removed on the following day, there was limited motion in one arm, which a doctor concluded could have resulted from either the child's struggle or the tightness of the restraint. The appellate court, in reversing a dismissal of the complaint, commented that a greater standard of care should be exercised in the treatment of the very young or very old, especially if they are under sedation or semiconscious.[91]

An unattended and unrestrained patient suffering from mental and emotional illness so seriously damaged both of her eyes as to make herself blind. A judgment for the hospital was given in a $150,000 damage suit since the court said that the objective of the hospitalization is treatment and restrictions must be kept at a minimum if the patient's confidence is to be restored.[92]

Even though a nursing restraint proved faulty for keeping an electroshock patient in bed after treatment, the patient could not recover for injuries when ties on a restraining sheet were tied in accordance with the recognized method of keeping a patient in bed after electroshock treatment and when the only standard of care established was used in treating and restraining the patient. The patient, who was suffering from depression and schizo-affective disorder, was receiving Glissando therapy, a part of which is electroshock therapy and restraint of the patient for four to five hours. The patient broke her hip when she fell out of bed.[93]

STERILIZATION

Sterilization is a procedure which renders the individual unable to produce offspring. As a voluntary procedure, it has received increased attention in recent years, partly because certain private and governmental agencies advocate birth control to limit the size of families. Except in Connecticut, Virginia, North Carolina, Georgia, Kansas and Utah, there are no state laws regulating voluntary sterilization. Moreover, there are no case decisions declaring voluntary sterilization illegal or against public policy. In Connecticut, Kansas and Utah, therapeutic or eugenic sterilization is permitted, but for anyone else it is a crime. Both Virginia and North Carolina have requirements for the consent of the spouse, parent or guardian and also for consultation, hospitalization and a waiting period. By an act of the 1966 General Assembly, physicians in Georgia who perform voluntary sterilization surgery have immunity from criminal and civil suits.

In voluntary nontherapeutic sterilization, physicians have been warned by the A.M.A. to obtain the consent of the patient's spouse because of the legal argument that husband and wife have a mutual interest in each other's ability to procreate. Also, Howard Hassard, counsel for the California Medical Association, has advised physicians against performing a sterilization until the law is more definitive:

> ... except when it is therapeutically indicated or in accordance with a statute.[94]

In a case in which a man had a vasectomy performed because the couple wanted no more children, and afterward his wife became pregnant and they had another child, he sued the physician for breach of contract for money damages to rear and educate the child. The Pennsylvania Court held that to allow such damages would be against public policy.[95]

In *Christensen v. Thornby*,[96] a vasectomy was performed on the husband since further pregnancies would endanger the wife's health; it was not against public policy and the court's opinion seems to indicate that consent alone is sufficient.

Eugenic sterilization to prevent procreation of the unfit, such as the feeble-minded, mentally ill, habitual criminals and sexual deviates, is provided in more than half of the states: Maine, New Hampshire, Vermont, Connecticut, Delaware, Virginia, West Virginia, North Carolina, South Carolina, Georgia, Alabama, Mississippi, Indiana, Michigan, Wisconsin, Minnesota, North Dakota, South Dakota, Iowa, Kansas, Nebraska, Oklahoma, Montana, Utah, Idaho, Oregon, California and Arizona.

In therapeutic sterilization, the whole or an important part of the reproductive system is removed in order to preserve the life or health of the patient. If the surgery is performed after consultation with another physician or specialist and with the consent of the person (and, if the patient is married, the consent of the spouse), few lawsuits arise. However, medical men do not always agree on the grounds for therapeutic sterilization. Surgery to reduce the spread of cancer in the breast or prostate gland is almost universally accepted, but there is great difference of opinion as to whether, say, inactive tuberculosis or mild diabetes is a proper ground for therapeutic sterilization.

Aside from the law, there are moral and religious objections to contraceptive sterilization, and if such operations are permissible in a hospital or doctor's office and the physician is willing to perform them, the religious convictions of patients should not be disregarded.

Roman Catholic View

The Roman Catholic Church has stated:

> Direct sterilization, namely the practice that aims to make procreation impossible, is a grave violation of moral law and therefore illicit.

If a pathological condition of the organ renders it necessary for the preservation of the patient's life and health, sterilization of a female is licit. If the purpose of the operation is to prevent the inconvenience or dangers of child bearing, it is illicit.[97] A hysterectomy is permitted only if the pathology of the patient warrants it. Removal of the ovaries, or oophorectomy, for the prevention of metastasis or in the treatment of cancer of the breast is permissible upon consultation and prudent medical advice; the purpose is to prevent spread of the disease, not contraception.[98] Similarly, when no less drastic and equally effective procedure is reasonably available, orchidectomy may be done when it offers some hope of benefit, as long as the purpose is not contraception.[99] Vasectomy should not be performed unless there is sufficient medical reason.

The Roman Catholic Church opposes eugenic sterilization of the mentally defective and physically diseased as a mutilation of a person guilty of no crime and one whom the state should not punish because of his misfortune.[100] The licitness of punitive sterilization performed on criminals as a penalty for their crimes is disputed by moralists. Again, Healy points out that it seems to be illicit to sterilize criminals for sex crimes because it leaves the sex organs otherwise intact and hence encourages rather than deters the sex offender in his crime.[101]

WRONGFUL DEATH

A number of civil actions are brought to recover damages for wrongful death if a statute permits such action. For example, parents brought an action to recover for the wrongful death of an 8½-year-old child who was mentally and physically unable to care for himself. The child's condition was known to an attendant, who nevertheless was negligent in her attention; as a result the child was scalded when he fell into a bathtub of hot water while he was an inmate at a state institution. The child died from burns after four days. The parents recovered damages for the child's personal suffering and for funeral expenses.[102]

There are a number of other civil actions brought to recover damages following gross negligence, abortion, apparently aggravated assault, and so forth. Actions of this nature will be discussed later in connection with crime (Chap. Nine). It should be mentioned that civil action for damages may arise from a wrongful death.

AUTOPSY PROCEEDINGS

When a patient dies, it is often necessary from a legal standpoint, or desirable from an informational or learning standpoint, to do an autopsy. The nurse should know something about this subject. There is no right of property in a corpse.[103] An autopsy is the dissection of a dead body for the purpose of inquiring into the cause of death. In general, a person has a right to dispose of his own body, and the laws and decisions tend to uphold his desires. A patient's surviving spouse, children, next-of-kin or friends are generally entitled to receive the corpse intact for the purpose of burial. Unless there is a statutory exception or consent, any willful mutilation of a patient's body, such as an autopsy, gives rise to an action for damages.

Generally speaking, a person will not be penalized if he in good faith secures consent for an autopsy from a relative or other person who appears to be responsible for the burial of the body. The nurse is reminded that more than once there has been a legal dispute over just who is entitled to the dead body. Persons entitled to a dead body include the surviving spouse, an adult child, parent or guardian, or the nearest relative or friends. However, such persons are not necessarily consulted in this order. For example, a person who has taken no interest in a patient during his lifetime could hardly be expected to be consulted when the patient died. More often than not, the first person sought is a relative with whom the patient lived. Generally, at the time of admission to a hospital, a patient is required to list his next-of-kin. It is reasonable that hospital personnel, including nurses, should accept such a person and not be expected to look elsewhere.

With respect to a dead body, an operation generally accepted by custom is legal. The work of embalmers and the customary postmortem examinations made by members of the medical profession for medical and scientific purposes are legal, provided due consideration is given to provisions in the will of the deceased or the desires of his next-of-kin.

In cases of deaths from violence or suspicious circumstances, at common law a coroner was required to hold an inquest and seek evidence to prevent a wrongdoer's escaping justice.[104] To determine whether a death is caused by natural or other means, the coroner may perform an autopsy. Today in many states the reporting of cases to a coroner or medical examiner is governed by statutory law. Some of the deaths which commonly must be reported include those due to suicide, homicide, abortion, accident, deaths occurring after a patient's being under doctor's care or in a hospital for a short time, deaths that are unexpected and those that are likely to be followed by criminal action. The coroner or medical examiner has the right to determine whether he will do an autopsy, and he can do so without the consent of the patient's spouse, next-of-kin, or friends.[105]

An insurance company may request to examine the body of an insured person and, if not forbidden by law, may do an autopsy to determine whether death was a result of any cause excluded from coverage under its contract with the insured. However, unless an insurance company secures a valid consent, it has no standing at law to demand an autopsy.

By way of illustration, a case in the Denver General Hospital may remind the nurse of what may happen. Two men in adjoining beds died at about the same time. A nurse, following the usual custom, prepared death tags, but through mistake or negligence attached a tag prepared for the other man to the body of the plaintiff's husband. The other man's family gave consent for an autopsy, and as a result of the nurse's error in tags the body of the plaintiff's husband was sent to the morgue and an autopsy performed. The plaintiff sued the hospital, hospital manager, coroner and pathologist for damages for the unauthorized autopsy. The pathologist was held not liable under the circumstances, since he proceeded with due care and without wrong intent on the basis of the information as usually supplied. The hospital as a governmental institution was immune. The hospital manager and coroner were not associated with this particular autopsy.[106] The nurse whose negligent actions were the proximate cause of the dispute was not sued in this action. However, the case illustrates how a nurse may incur liability to suit, and it confirms the need of exercising reasonable care in all her work.

TRANSPLANTATION OF ORGANS

Cardiac transplantation, often presented as a tense and emotional drama by the various mass media of communication, has stimulated the public to think about the legal and ethical problems involved. As a result, the archaic and cumbersome laws controlling the disposition of the body and its various parts came to light, and essential reform has been undertaken. To date, 44 jurisdictions, including the District of Columbia, have enacted donation statutes which enable an adult to donate all or part of his body for medical, therapeutic or scientific purposes. In Maine, West Virginia, Georgia and Alaska, this donation is restricted to the eyes. As yet, New Hampshire, Vermont and Utah have no donation statute.[107] Although these donation statutes have eliminated some of the uncertainties and problems, in the main, they are inadequate as measured by current needs. The Commissioners on Uniform State Laws have made important advances in preparing the Uniform Anatomical Gift Act, which eliminates the chief legal constraints without compromising other important rights and sensitivities.[108] This Act was approved by the Commissioners on July 30, 1968, and was endorsed a week later by the American Bar Association on August 7, 1968.

This Uniform Anatomical Gift Act solves a number of problems: Section 2(a) provides that any person of sound mind and 18 years of age or more may give his body or any part of it for purposes listed in the act, Sections 3, 4(c) and (d) and the gift to become effective after death. Under English common law, the next-of-kin had the right to possession of the body for burial, so the person had no say in the disposal of his body.[109] Furthermore, since the next-of-kin are the ones who have control over the dead body, Section 2(b) gives them authority to donate the body or a part thereof, and, to resolve possible disagreements, provides an order of priority among them. Section 2(e) provides the wish of the donor control if there is a difference between the donor's plans and those of relatives, while Section 2(d) permits whatever examination is needed to ascertain whether the proposed gift is medically acceptable for use. Section 7(b) provides:

> The time of death shall be determined by a physician who attends the donor at his death, or, if none, the physician who certifies the death. This physician shall not participate in the proceedings for removing or transplanting a part.

Section 7(c) protects all persons, including physicians, from liability in civil and criminal actions. However, the Act does not purport to decide other problems, such as the time of death and criteria for selecting recipients, which are the work of allied disciplines.[110] The adoption of this Act has been supported by the American Medical Association, American Heart Association, the Eye Banks Association of America, The National Kidney Foundation and many other organizations.

The initial guidelines that we have to protect the patient and physicians were developed during the Nuremburg Trials which followed World War II when the public was shocked by the experimentation carried out by Nazi physicians. Growing out of that situation was the Declaration of Helsinki, which contains recommendation for the guidance of doctors in clinical research, and it was adopted by the World Medical Association in 1964. The basic principles set forth in that Declaration are:

> 1. Clinical research must conform to the moral and scientific principles that justify medical research and should be based on laboratory and animal experiments or other scientifically established facts.

2. Clinical research should be conducted only by scientifically qualified persons and under the supervision of a qualified medical man.

3. Clinical research cannot legitimately be carried out unless the importance of the objective is in proportion to the inherent risk to the subject.

4. Every clinical research project should be preceded by careful assessment of inherent risks in comparison to foreseeable benefits to the subjects or to others.

5. Special caution should be exercised by the doctor in performing clinical research in which the personality of the subject is liable to be altered by drugs or experimental procedure.[111]

An editorial in the *New England Journal of Medicine* states:

The principles involved are, in substance, that the subject of an experiment involving any risk must stand to benefit by it; that his informed consent must be obtained to the fullest degree possible; finally and more important than any specific rules that have yet been devised, the investigator must be "intelligent, informed, conscientious, compassionate, responsible."[112]

The time of death is the subject of much discussion and many articles. Black's *Law Dictionary*[113] defines death as:

The cessation of life; the ceasing to exist; defined by physicians as the total stoppage of the circulation of blood, and a cessation of the animal and vital functions consequent thereupon, such as respiration, pulsation, etc.

In two recent cases, this definition was used.[114] More recently, the definition of irreversible coma, formulated by a committee at the Harvard Medical School, gives these characteristics: (1) unreceptivity and unresponsitivity, (2) no movements of breathing, (3) no reflexes and (4) flat electroencephalogram.[115] The statement on death by the Twenty-second World Medical Assembly in Sydney, Australia, in August, 1968, states that the determination of the time of death is and should remain the legal responsibility of the physician.[116] It points out that two modern procedures have made further study of the question of the time of death necessary; viz., the ability to maintain by artificial means the circulation of oxygenated blood through tissues of the body which have been irreversibly injured, and the use of cadavers' organs for transplants. Furthermore, it states that if transplantation of an organ is involved, the decision that the donor is dead should be made by two or more physicians who are not connected with the transplantation procedure.

The question of whether to use extreme measures to prolong life has bothered and continues to bother people. Selected references on this topic will be found at the end of the chapter.[117] In general, it would seem, one is obliged to use ordinary means to preserve life, but the use of extraordinary means to prolong life is not obligatory.

Transplants of kidneys, corneas, skin and bone have been done many times, and some with a fairly high degree of success, without causing the mind-searching engendered by heart transplants. The number of heart and liver transplants has been limited, and the problem differs from, say, kidney transplantation in that death is inevitable for the donor. However, when the kidney transplant involves the removal of one kidney from a living donor, we have the question of the risk of serious complications or death to a living donor, and must ask whether the results of surgery using living donors is sufficiently good to justify injuring a healthy person to improve the well-being of another.[118] The degree of success of renal transplants coupled with the minute decrease in the donor's life expectancy is suggested as justifying the renal transplant procedure.[119] However, the thorny problem of "Who among us is to decide who will be donor and who a recipient?" remains.

In *Sirianni v. Anna*,[120] the plaintiff voluntarily donated a kidney to her son, who needed it to save his life. She alleged that malpractice occurred in the removal of her son's kidney. Although the son survived and his claim for damages was settled, the mother still sued the surgeon, claiming that her own health had been impaired by the unnecessary loss of her donated kidney. The court did not permit the mother to recover.

In the matter of transplants, it is interesting to note that the Internal Revenue Service Ruling 68-452 provides that a donor's travel, medical and hospital expense are deductible medical expenses of the recipient if he pays for them.

A brief word concerning the ethical aspects seems necessary. The American Medical Association has published *Ethical Guidelines for Organ Transplantation*.[121] One prominent Presbyterian minister has said:

> There are no moral or ethical implications involved in an actual organ transplant.[122]

The view of S. S. Kety is:

> The moral obligation of performing all human experiments, with due regard to the sensibility, welfare, and safety of the subject, must not be violated. As phrased by Claude Bernard in 1856, "Christian morals forbid only one thing, doing ill to one's neighbor." So, among experiments that may be tried on man, those that can do only harm are forbidden, those that are harmless are permissible, and those that may do good are obligatory.[123]

Concerning organ transplantation among the living, Lowery points out that there are two schools of thought. One group holds that transplantation of organs among the living is immoral, and their reasoning is:

> Man is the only administrator of his life and bodily functions; his power to dispose of these things is limited. He can allow

serious self-mutilation when it is for the good of his own person, because that is reasonable administration. But he cannot allow serious self-mutilation for the benefit of another person.[124]

He also points out that a second school of thought holds that organ transplantation among the living

> ... is morally justifiable provided it confers a proportionate benefit on the recipient, without exposing the donor to a greater risk or depriving him completely of an important function.[125]

This brief citation of the ethical views of various men is intended merely to show the reader that there is a considerable variety and diversity of opinion among sincere men upon this topic.

REFERENCES

1. Prosser: *Torts,* 3rd ed. 1964, § 1, 2 Baudry-Lacantinerie: *Précis de droit civil,* 7th ed. par. 1346-7. Lee: Torts and Delicts. 27 *Yale L.J.* 721 (1928). *Salmond on the Law of Torts,* 9th ed., 1936. § 3-5
2. *Restatement, Torts.* § 281
3. Clark: *Law of Code Pleading,* 2nd ed. 1947. §§ 13, 64
4. Prosser: *op. cit. supra.* note 1, § 10. Carpenter: Intentional Invasions of Interest in Personality. 13 *Ore. L. Rev.* 227, 275 (1934)
5. Pollock: *Torts,* 14th ed. 1939, p. 170; Miller: *Criminal Law.* Hornbook, 1936, 101; Assault and Battery, Civil Liability 1(b), 6 C.J.S. 796
6. Prosser: *op. cit. supra.* note 1, § 18
7. O'Brien v. Cunard S.S. Co., 154 Mass. 272, 28 N.E. 266 (1891); 13 L.R.A. 329
8. Hughes, James J., Jr.: The Hospital, the Physician and Informed Consent. *Hospitals,* 42:66-70, June 16, 1968. This article contains a review and citation of a number of cases
9. Luka v. Lowrie, 171 Mich. 122, 136 N.W. 1106 (1912)
10. Jackovach v. Yocom, 212 Iowa 914, 237 N.W. 444 (1931)
11. Wells v. McGhee, 39 So. 2d 196, (La., 1949)
12. Zoski v. Gaines, 271 Mich. 1, 260 N.W. 99 (1935)
13. Bakkar v. Welsh, 144 Mich. 632, 108 N.W. 94 (1906)
14. Lacey v. Laird, 166 Ohio 12, 139 N.E. 2d 25 (1956)
15. Russell, Donald H.: Law, Medicine and Minors. *New Eng. J. Med.,* 278:779-80, Apr. 4, 1968. Brown, H. G.: Parental Right to Refuse Medical Treatment for Child. *Crime and Delinquency,* 12(4) 377-85, Oct., 1966
16. *Idem.*
17. Laws of Maryland, Ch. 468, Sec. 1 (1968)
18. Massachusetts General Laws, Ch. 1, Sec. 117 (1954); Connecticut, Public Act No. 206 (1968). See Russell, Donald H.: Law, Medicine, and Minors, Part I. *New Eng. J. Med.,* 278:35-36, Jan. 4, 1968
19. Brooks Estate v. Brooks, 32 Ill. 2d 361, 205 N.E. 2d 435 (1965)
20. Regan, William A.: O.R. Nursing and Unorthodox Surgery. *Regan Report on Nursing Law,* 7(5) 1, Oct., 1966
21. Fiorentino v. Wenger, 26 A.D. 2d 693 272 N.Y.S. 2d 557 (1966)
22. Barbee, Grace C.: Consents: the Nurse's Role in Obtaining and Using Them. *Hospital Forum,* 9:23-24, Sept., 1966
23. Lear, John: Experiments on People—The Growing Debate. *Saturday Review,* July 2, 1966, pp. 41-43
24. Clarke, Alice R.: (*editorial*) Patient Consent in Research. *Nurs. Forum,* VI (1) 10-11, 118, 1967. See also Downs, Florence S.: Ethical Inquiry in Nursing Research. *Nurs. Forum,* VI (1) 12-20, 1967
25. Cancer-Implant Test Brings Threat of Million Dollar Suit for Damages. *The Physician's Legal Brief,* Bloomfield, Shering Corp., 1964

26. Prosser: *op. cit. supra.* note 1, § 19. See also Perkins: Self-defense Re-examined. 1 *U.S.C.L.A. Rev.* 133 (1954)
27. Commonwealth v. Gregory, 132 Pa. Super. 507 (1911)
28. Wood v. Wyeth, 106 App. Div. 21, 81 N.Y.S. 1148, 94 N.Y.S. 361 (1905)
29. Beaucoudray v. Hirsch, 49 So. 2d 770 (Ct. of Appeals of La., 1951). See also this subject in 6 C.J.S. 807
30. Main v. Ellsworth, 237 Iowa 970, 23 N.W. 2d 429 (1946).
31. Martin v. Carbide & Carbon Chemicals Corp. *et al.,* 184 Tenn. 166, 197 S.W. 2d 798 (1946)
32. Prosser: *op. cit. supra.* note 1, § 20
33. Prosser: *op. cit. supra.* note 1, § 21
34. Beale: Justification for Injury. 41 *Harvard L. Rev.* 553 (1928)
35. Prosser: *op. cit. supra.* note 1, § 8. Hall: Interrelations of Criminal Law and Torts. 43 *Col. L. Rev.* 753, 967 (1943)
36. Burrows v. Hawaiian Trust Co., 49 Hawaii Rep. 351, 417 P.2d 816 (1966)
37. Nelson v. Rural Educational Assn. *et al.,* 23 Tenn. App. 409, 134 S.W. 2d 181 (1939)
38. Sarlat v. State of New York, 52 Misc. 2d 240, 275 N.Y.S. 2d 293 (1966)
39. 384 U.S. 757 (1966). See also discussion by Hershey, Nathan: When Police Ask for a Blood Sample. *Am. J. Nursing,* 68:540-1, March, 1968, which points out that the decision does not necessarily prevent an action for battery
40. Kan. Stat. Ann. § 8-1001 (Supp. 1967)
41. N.Y. Law Ch. 615 (1966)
42. See *The Child Abuse Reporting Laws.* Washington, D.C., Children's Bureau, U.S. Dept. of Health, Education and Welfare, 1966. Foster, Henry H.: The Battered Child. *Am. Trial Lawyers,* Dec.-Jan., 1966-67, pp. 33-7. Kempe, Henry C.: The Battered Child Syndrome. *J.A.M.A.,* 181:17-24, July 7, 1962. Child-abuse Laws in the 50 States. *RN,* 31:67-68, Dec., 1968; Mississippi Child Abuse Law Covers Reporting Nurses. *Am. J. Nursing,* 67:15, Jan., 1967
43. In the Matter of S., 259 N.Y.S. 2d 164 (Fam. Ct., 1965)
44. Paulsen, Monrad G.: Legal Protections Against Child Abuse. *Children,* 13:43-48, Mar.-Apr., 1966
45. Cheney, Kimberly B.: Safeguarding Legal Rights in Providing Protective Services. *Children,* 13:87-92, May-June, 1966
46. *In re* Dubin, 112 N.Y.S. 2d 267 (1952)
47. Murphy v. Murphy, 143 Conn. 600, 124 A. 2d. 891 (1956)
48. Hunter v. Powers, 135 N.Y.S. 2d 371 (1954)
49. Savery v. Eddy, 242 Iowa 822, 45 N.W. 2d (1951)
50. State v. Greer, 311 S.W. 2d 49 (Mo., 1958)
51. Cheney: *op. cit. supra.* note 1
52. School Nurses' Responsibilities Viewed. *CNA Bull.,* 63:7, June, 1967
53. State of Washington v. Parmenter, 444 P.2d 680 (Wash., 1968)
54. Prosser: *op. cit. supra.* note 1, § 12. Harper: Malicious Prosecution, False Imprisonment, and Defamation. 15 *Tex. L. Rev.* 156 (1937)
55. Gadsden General Hospital v. Hamilton, 212 Ala. 531, 103 So. 553 (1925). See also Analysis of Legal and Medical Considerations in Commitment of the Mentally Ill. 56 *Yale L.J.* 1178 (1947)
56. Salisbury v. Poulson, 51 Utah 552, 172 Pac. 315 (1918)
57. Bailie v. Miami Valley Hospital, 221 N.E. 2d 217 (Ct. of Common Pleas, Ohio, 1966)
58. Whitree v. State of New York, 290 N.Y.S. 2d 486 (1968)
59. Ex-MU-Student Says She Was Imprisoned. *Milwaukee Journal,* Part 2, August 5, 1969, p. 9
60. 88 S. Ct. 2145 (Tex., 1968)
61. Zebell v. Krall, 348 Mich. 482, 83 N.W. 2d 288 (1957)
62. Niger: The Right of Privacy; a Half Century's Developments. 39 *Mich. L. Rev.* 526 (1941). Ludwig: Peace of Mind in 48 Pieces v. Uniform Right of Privacy. 32 *Minn. L. Rev.* 734 (1948). Yankwich: The Right of Privacy. 27 *Notre Dame Law.* 499 (1952). *Restatement, Torts.* § 867 (1939)
63. Prosser: *op. cit. supra.* note 1, § 97
64. *Restatement, Torts.* § 867 (1939)

65. Bazemore *et al.* v. Savannah Hospital *et al.,* 171 Ga. 257, 155 S.E. 194 (1930)
66. De May v. Roberts, 46 Mich. 160, 9 N.W. 146 (1881): See contra: Carr v. Shifflette, 82 F 2d 874 (Cir. D.C., 1936)
67. Melvin v. Reid, 112 Cal. App. 285, 297 Pac. 91 (1931). See Yandwich: The Right of Privacy. 27 *Notre Dame Law.* 499, note 22 (1952) for similar cases in point
68. Prosser: *op. cit. supra.* note 1, § 92. *Restatement, Torts.* § 559. Holdsworth: Defamation in the Sixteenth and Seventeenth Centuries. 40 *L.Q. Rev.* 302, 397 (1924); 41 *L.Q. Rev.* 13 (1925). Carr and "The English Law of Defamation," 18 *L.Q. Rev.* 255, 388 (1902); Donnelly: History of Defamation. 1949 *Wis. L. Rev.* 99. Yankwich: Certainty in the Law of Defamation. 1. *U.S.C.L.A. Rev.* 163 (1954)
69. Alpin v. Morton, 21 Ohio St. 536 (1871)
70. Prosser: *op. cit. supra.* note 1, §§ 93-96. *Restatement, Torts.* § 568. Donnelly: Defamation by Radio: A Reconsideration. 34 *Iowa L. Rev.* 12 (1948), 1 *Duke B.J.* 218 (1951)
71. Prosser: *op. cit. supra.* note 1, §§ 93-96
72. I Russell: *Crimes,* 8th ed. 1923, p. 983
73. Farrell v. Kramer, 159 Maine 387, 35 A|2 218, 193 A. 2d 560 (1963)
74. Prosser: *op. cit. supra.* note 1, § 95. Evans: Legal Immunity for Defamation. 24 *Minn. L. Rev.* 607 (1940)
75. Prosser: *op. cit. supra.* note 1, § 95
76. 1, 3 Scott: *Trusts* (1939, 1954 Supp.) §§ 2.5, 495. 1 *Restatement, Trusts.* § 2(b); also § 170(1) (2). 1 *Restatement, Agency.* 1933, § 13 — Agent as a fiduciary
77. New Jersey Session Laws, C. 185 (N.J., July 19, 1968)
78. Massachusetts Session Laws, C. 418 (Mass., June 18, 1968)
79. Alexander v. Knight, 177 A. 2d 142 (Pa., 1962)
80. Boulware v. Boulware, 153 So. 2d 182 (La., 1964)
81. Cleveland v. Maddox, 152 Ark. 538, 239 S.W. 370 (1922)
82. Culver v. Union P.R. Co., 112 Neb. 441, 199 N.W. 794 (1924)
83. Meyer v. Russell, 55 N.D. 546, 214 N.W. 857 (1927)
84. Hobbs v. Hullman, 183 App. Div. 743, 171 N.Y.S. 390 (1918) Judgment reversed for other error
85. Louisville & N.R. Co. v. Crockett's Adm'x., 232 Ky. 662, 24 S.W. 2d 580 (1930)
86. Dyer v. State, 241 Ala. 679, 4 So. 2d 311 (1941)
87. Flower's Case, Cro. Car., 211, 79 Eng. Rep. 785 (1632)
88. Amick v. Montross, 206 Iowa 51, 220 N.W. 51 (1928)
89. Rickbeil v. Grafton Deaconess Hospital *et al.,* 74 N.D. 525, 23 N.W. 2d 247 (1946)
90. Regan, William A.: Nursing Liability for Restraint Accidents. *Regan Report on Nursing Law,* 8(6) 1, Nov., 1967
91. Moore v. Halifax Hospital, 202 So. 2d 568 (Fla.)
92. Gerba v. Neurological Hospital, 1967 CCH Neg. 1660 (Mo.)
93. Constant v. Howe, 436 S.W. 2d 115 (Tex.)
94. Legal Risks Involved in Sterilization Cited by California Lawyer. *The Physician's Legal Brief,* 9(4) 3, April, 1967
95. Shaheen v. Knight, 6 N.Y.C. 19, 11 Pa. D&C. 2d 41 (1957)
96. Christensen v. Thornby, 192 Minn. 123, 255 N.W. 620 (1934)
97. Healy, Edwin F., S.J.: *Medical Ethics.* Chicago, Loyola University Press, 1956
98. *Idem.*
99. *Idem.*
100. *Idem.*
101. *Idem.*
102. Johnsen v. State, 176 Misc. 347, 27 N.Y.S. 2d 945 (1941)
103. Prosser: *op. cit. supra.* note 1, §§ 11, 37. *Restatement, Torts.* § 868. Fryer: Readings on Personal Property, 3rd ed. 1. Recent Case Notes. 9 *Ind. L.J.* 177 (1933-34)
104. Polk County v. Phillips, 92 Tex. 630, 51 S.W. 328 (1899)
105. Young v. College of Physicians and Surgeons, 81 Md. 358, 32 Atl. 177 (1895); 31 L.R.A. 540. See 10 Cent. L.J. 303 on disposal of dead body
106. Schwalb v. Connely, 116 Colo. 195, 179 P 2d 667 (1947). See also Hasselbach v. Mt. Sinai Hosp., 173 App. Div. 89, 159 N.Y.S. 376 (1916)
107. Sadler, A. M., Jr., and Sadler, B. L.: Transplantation and Law: Need for Organized Sensitivity. *Georgetown Law J.* 57:5-54, 1968
108. Sadler, A. M., Jr., Sadler, B. L. and Stason, E. B.: Uniform Anatomical Gift Act;

Model for Reform. *J.A.M.A.,* 206:2501-6, 1968. Curran, W. J.: Law-Medicine Notes: Uniform Anatomical Gift Act. *New Eng. J. Med.,* 280:36, 1969

109. Stason, E. B.: Role of Law in Medical Progress. *Law & Contemp. Prob.,* 32:563-596, 1967

110. Stickel, D. L.: Ethical and Moral Aspects of Transplantation. *Monogr. in Surg. Sc.,* 3:267-301, 1966. Report of the Ad Hoc Committee of the Harvard Medical School to Examine the Definition of Brain Death; a Definition of Brain Death. *J.A.M.A.,* 205:337-340, Aug. 5, 1968

111. Wolstenholme, G. E. W., and O'Connor, M. (eds.): *Ciba Foundation Symposium: Ethics in Medical Progress, with Special Reference to Transplantation.* Boston, Little, Brown & Co., 1966

112. Experimentation in Man. (editorial.) *New Eng. J. Med.,* 274:1382-3, June 16, 1966

113. *Black's Law Dictionary,* 4th ed. 1951

114. Thomas v. Anderson, 96 Cal. App. 2d 371 (1950). Smith v. Smith, 229 Ark. 579, 317 S.W.2d 275 (1958)

115. Report of the Ad Hoc Committee of the Harvard Medical School to Examine the Definition of Brain Death; a Definition of Irreversible Coma. *J.A.M.A.,* 205:337-340, Aug. 5, 1968

116. Quoted in Wecht, Cyril: Attorney Describes Current Efforts to Establish Uniform Guidelines (in death and transplantation). *Hospitals,* 43:54-7, Nov. 1, 1969

117. Fletcher, G. P.: Legal Aspects of the Decision Not to Prolong Life. *J.A.M.A.,* 203:65-8, Jan. 1, 1968. Whitlow, B., *et al.*: Extreme Measures to Prolong Life. *J.A.M.A.,* 202:374-6, Oct. 23, 1967. Armiger, B.: About Questioning the Right to Die; Reprise and Dialogue. *Nurs. Outlook,* 16:26-8, Oct., 1968. Whitlow, the Very Rev. Brian (Episcopalian): Extreme Measures to Prolong Life. *J.A.M.A.,* 202:226-7, Oct. 23, 1967. Healy, Edwin F., S. J.: Means That Must Be Used to Preserve Life. *Medical Ethics.* Chicago, Loyola Univ. Press, 1956, pp. 60-90. Levy, J. S.: The Patient—The Physician—The Clergy—The Challenge. *J. Arkansas Med. Soc.,* 64:162, Sept., 1967. Williamson, W. P., *et al.*: Prolongation of Life or Prolonging the Act of Dying. *J.A.M.A.,* 202:162-3, Oct. 9, 1967. Bronstein, R. H.: Heart Transplants: Three Views: The Power Over Life and Death. *Dis. Chest,* 54:346-8, Oct., 1968

118. Conn, Julius, Jr.: Difficulty in Establishing Goals for Clinical Efforts. *Hospitals,* 43:49-50, Nov. 1, 1969

119. *Idem.*

120. 285 N.Y.S. 2d 709 (Sup. Ct. of Niag. City., 1967)

121. Ethical Guidelines for Organ Transplantation. *J.A.M.A.,* 205:341-2, Aug. 5, 1968

122. McCleave, Paul, D. D.: Clergyman Says "Moral Problems" Stem From Emotions, Not Ethics. *Hospitals,* 43:53-4, Nov. 1, 1969

123. Page, I. H.: The Ethics of Heart Transplants. *J.A.M.A.,* 207:109-13, Jan. 6, 1969

124. Lowery, Daniel L.: Questions about Organ Transplants. *Liguorian,* 56(3)12-15, Mar., 1968

125. *Idem.*

Chapter Nine

Crimes: Misdemeanors and Felonies

Nurses, like other citizens, may subject themselves to criminal prosecution either by doing something which the law defines as a criminal act or by omitting to do an act which the law requires and the omission of which the law declares to be a crime. Moreover, a person does not have to do something immoral or wicked for the law to regard the act as criminal. For example, if a state, using its police power, makes it mandatory for all nurses who practice nursing for hire to obtain a license, and provides that willful violation of such law shall constitute a misdemeanor, then a nurse who renders nursing service for pay without securing a license is guilty of a crime, even though she may not intend to do wrong. Again, some acts of negligence are so gross or wanton in character as to be classified as crimes.

DEFINITION OF CRIMINAL ACTIONS

Criminal actions deal with acts or offenses against the public welfare. These are considered offenses against the state and vary from minor, petty offenses and misdemeanors to felonies. A misdemeanor is a general name for every sort of criminal offense which

169

does not in law amount to the grade of felony. A felony in many states is defined as any public offense for the conviction of which a person is liable to be sentenced to death or to imprisonment in a penitentiary or state prison.[1] A felony implies that the crime has more serious consequences or is of a more atrocious nature than a misdemeanor.

Every adult person of sound mind recognizes the acts of murder, rape, manslaughter, robbery and larceny as crimes. Likewise, assault may be a criminal offense as well as the basis of a tort action for damages, as may most crimes.

Certain wrongs are identified as crimes because they are regarded as harmful to public health, welfare, safety or security. In the last analysis, public policy or the will of the people as expressed by law determines what shall be classified as criminal wrong. In our country, by virtue of the police power, Congress has the power to decide which wrongs are crimes in federal matters, and each state legislature has the power to declare what wrongs will be classified as crimes within its jurisdiction. Because public policy as expressed by law determines the category of crimes, acts which are criminal in one country may not be so in another. As a society or state grows, the pressure to express its standards of social conduct in law increases.

REQUIREMENTS FOR CONVICTION

Criminal offenses are composed of two elements; a criminal act and a criminal intent. In order to convict a person of a crime, both must be proved beyond a reasonable doubt. A criminal offense is either some act which the law forbids or the omission of some act which the law requires.

Criminal intent is the state of mind a person has at the time that the criminal act is committed; this means knowing that an act is not lawful and deciding to do it anyway. To be criminal, an act must be defined as a crime by law. When there is an actual doing of a criminal act, the courts, except in specific intent crimes, presume a criminal intent unless the person who is accused of the crime attempts to show that at the time such criminal action was committed it was an involuntary act or that he was not capable of understanding or deciding the essential character of the act and its unlawful nature. To prove the same, he may offer evidence showing insanity, necessity, compulsion, accident, infancy, or mistake of fact. Although an act may be recognized as criminal, nevertheless, if a person is able to prove to the satisfaction of the court the lack of criminal intent due to one or more of the conditions cited, the court will decide he did not commit a criminal offense and will declare the person not guilty. In other words, although the law may presume intent upon the doing of a particular act, it cannot presume intent on the part of persons who are incapable of it.[2]

ARGUMENTS AGAINST CRIMINAL INTENT

Insanity

As a defense to a crime in criminal law, insanity has been defined as such a deranged condition of the mental and moral faculties as to make a person incapable of knowing whether his acts are right or wrong.[3] Statutes have been passed in a number of states providing for medical examination of an accused person when there is a question concerning his sanity. Experts are often requested to examine the accused person and to testify during the trial as to a person's sanity at the time of examination and also to speculate as to his mental state when the crime was committed. In some states, in addition to the "right and wrong test," there is an "irresistible impulse test."[4] An irresistible impulse is symptomatic of mental disease which causes a person to commit an act despite his ability to differentiate between right and wrong. As pointed out in the discussion of contracts, where it was mentioned that an insane person could not make a valid contract, the whole problem of whether or not a person is insane is many times difficult to determine. However difficult insanity may be to ascertain, an insane person cannot be legally charged with criminal intent.[5]

Necessity or Compulsion

Necessity is a defense to a charge of criminal intent and action. There are occasions when a nurse must defend herself from attack and bodily harm by a violent patient. If she is able to prove that in defending herself she used only the force necessary to repel the attack, she is not guilty of criminal intent, despite the injuries inflicted upon her assailant.

Accident

If an act is an accident, this might relieve one of criminal intent. For example, assume that a nurse was out playing golf, and she hit a ball which, after striking a tree, bounced off, striking a child and seriously injuring his eye. The nurse did nothing a reasonable person would not do in the circumstances, and yet an accident resulted; the injury was due neither to criminal intent nor to gross negligence.

Mistake of Fact

Suppose a hospital pharmacy put up boric acid solution and dextrose solution in similar bottles, similarly labeled, except that on the boric acid bottle label it said "For external use only." Assume further that newborn babies were customarily fed 5 per cent dextrose solution. Assume, too, that a druggist's helper mistakenly filled a dextrose bottle with boric acid and a nurse fed the solution to several babies and they died.[6] The nurse would not be responsible for their deaths. Her action, due to a mistake of fact, lacked criminal intent.

Infancy

Moreover, the law recognizes that criminal intent may be absent because of a person's infancy. Though children may be convicted of crimes, as a general rule children under 7 years are conclusively presumed to be unable to differentiate criminal right and wrong in the legal sense. Hence, if a 5-year-old who was at times jealous of his baby sister fed her 10 pink aspirin tablets as "candy," and the sister was harmed thereby, it would be presumed that the little boy had entertained no criminal intention. Also, minors from 7 years to 14 years are in many states chargeable only with juvenile delinquency, not crime.

GROSS NEGLIGENCE

We have noted that ordinary negligence is not a crime. However, when the negligence is extremely careless or reckless, with disregard for human life, it becomes something more serious, namely, gross negligence. As has been stated, at least two elements are necessary for deliberate crime: evil intent and criminal action. There are crimes in which the matter of intent is not spelled out, such as some grossly negligent act and the person is ignorant of the law.

DISTINCTION BETWEEN CRIMINAL LIABILITY AND TORT

Criminal liability is to be distinguished from tort liability. In a criminal action, the state seeks the punishment of the wrongdoer. In a tort action, which is a civil action, the person who has been wronged seeks to be compensated for the injury or wrong he has suffered on account of the acts of the wrongdoer. The same set of circumstances, such as negligence causing the death of a person, may give rise to both a criminal action and a civil action, but these actions are tried in different courts with different procedures. In a criminal case, there is a heavy burden on the prosecution to prove its case beyond a reasonable doubt, whereas in a civil action all that the plaintiff has to do is to show a preponderance (excess of weight or influence) of evidence in his favor. Therefore, it may happen that a person may escape punishment for a crime and yet be liable in a civil suit arising out of the same event.

In a California case, under a statute which provided that when the death of a person is caused by a wrongful act of another, his heirs may maintain an action against the person causing the death, an administrator brought a civil suit against a private hospital, physician and head nurse for damages for a wrongful death. The deceased patient had been a cook who earned high wages and sent most of them to his mother in Italy. After some years, he decided to make a trip to Italy, and apparently became so excited and nervous about the trip that it was necessary to take him to a private hospital. The evidence tended to show that the patient was not violent, but that he was merely excitable and had sudden outbursts — a condition which frequently yields to rest and treatment. Evidence also established that the santiarium was equipped with restraining straps, which were not used, and that the patient's death resulted either from excessive use of ether or from the application of a tourniquet which consisted of a towel placed about his neck. There was considerable evidence concerning a violent struggle, that four or five persons were subduing him, and that most of the contents of a pound can of ether were used. The struggle lasted some time. A $15,000 award to a mother with a life expectancy of 13 years was held not excessive.[7] Though this is a civil action and no mention is made of a criminal action against the doctor and nurse, it illustrates the possibilities of a nurse as well as others rendering herself liable.

All criminal actions are brought in the name of the state, such as State versus Staples. By contrast, a civil action is, for example, Jennie Jones, plaintiff, versus Sue Smith, defendant. It is a principle of our law that in any legal action, "every person is entitled to his day in court," and it is hoped that the following brief summary of procedure at a criminal trial, in addition to the previous brief outline of the conduct of civil actions, will give the nurse some appreciation of how this right is secured for each person, both citizen and alien.

CRIMINAL COURT PROCEDURE

Briefly, the procedure at a criminal trial is as follows: The accused person is brought before the court, and the indictment or charges are read aloud. The office of the grand jury is to examine the basis on which a charge is made by the state.[8] After this, the accused person is asked whether he pleads guilty or not guilty. If he pleads guilty, and if the court is satisfied that the person knows full well the meaning of what he says, then it may sentence him. However, the court must, if it is a capital punishment offense, ignore a plea of guilty and enter a plea of not guilty. In any very serious case, the court may ignore the accused person's plea of guilty and enter a plea of not guilty. Under our criminal laws in the United States, a person is always presumed innocent until proved guilty beyond a reasonable doubt. In very serious cases, the court enters a plea of not guilty in an accused person's behalf, even when he pleads guilty, in order to put on the prosecutor the burden of proving him guilty beyond a reasonable doubt. When the accused person is thus arraigned (called before the court to answer to an indictment), preparations for the trial are made.

If it is a jury trial, the jurors are then selected and sworn in to give a true verdict. The prosecutor opens the trial with a statement in which he outlines the important features of the case; then the witnesses are called. A witness is examined, followed by cross-examination by the defense attorney for the accused. The witness may be re-examined by the prosecutor followed by a re-cross-examination. After the state's case has been presented, the attorney for the accused may request the court to dismiss the case and discharge the accused on the ground that no case has been made against him. If the court agrees, it directs the jury to return a verdict of not guilty; otherwise, the trial proceeds, and witnesses are called for the defense. They are examined by the defense attorney; then they may be cross-examined by the prosecutor, and again they may be re-examined by the defense. When all the defense has been heard, then the prosecutor and the defense attorney each address the jury in summation. The court then instructs the jury and asks them to consider their verdict. The jurors retire to a designated room to do so. If the accused person is found not guilty, he is discharged. If the accused person is found guilty, the presiding judge pronounces sentence. After a person has been tried on a criminal charge and either discharged or convicted, he may not be tried on that same charge again by the same sovereign. If a person is tried in a lower court, he may, as a rule, appeal to a higher court if he can show some error in the proceedings.

LEGAL TERMS: FELONY AND MISDEMEANOR

A brief review of certain legal terms follows, with a view to clarifying their meaning for the nurse. A felony at common law was an offense which brought about a total forfeiture of either a person's land or goods, or both, and to which capital or other punishment might be added according to the degree of guilt. In American law, the word "felony" has no clear, definite meaning at common law, but it includes offenses of considerable gravity. A crime is not a felony unless it is so declared by statute or it was so at common law.[10] In the United States Criminal Code,[11] all offenses that are punishable by death, by imprisonment for one year or more, or by a fine in excess of $1000 are felonies; all other offenses are misdemeanors. For example, if a nurse were convicted of performing an illegal abortion, that act would be a felony. On the other hand, if a nurse were convicted of unlawfully taking a three-dollar bottle of wine from a patient's locker, that would be a misdemeanor.

MORAL TURPITUDE

A person sometimes hears or sees the words "moral turpitude." That term refers to an act of baseness, vileness or depravity in social and private duties.[12] Crimes involving moral turpitude are acts which are bad in themselves, such as rape, robbery and murder.

MURDER

Murder is the unlawful killing of a human being with intent to kill. In every case, murder is a very serious crime, the penalty for which may be death, life imprisonment or a lesser punishment. There can be no consent to killing a person. In passing, it seems instructive to remind nurses that in our country euthanasia (an act or practice of painlessly putting to death persons suffering from incurable or distressing disease) is murder according to our law.[9] Also, a death occurring as a result of an illegal abortion is murder.

Homicide and Murder

Sometimes nurses use the words "homicide" and "murder" interchangeably, but they have different meanings. Homicide is the killing of one human being by another, and it may be justifiable, excusable, or a felony.[13] The homicide is regarded as justifiable in executing a death sentence, in suppressing a riot, in preventing a felony, and, in some cases, in defending oneself, one's home or others.[14] An example of an excusable homicide would be a killing done in necessary, reasonable self-defense or by an unavoidable accident.[15]

On the other hand, murder, properly speaking, is the unlawful killing of one human being by another with "malice aforethought."[16] Malice aforethought indicates purpose and design in a person's action, in contrast to accident. To exhibit malice aforethought, a person does not necessarily have to intend to kill another or to do it deliberately, but in general, it is enough if, at the time that the crime was done, the person intended serious bodily harm or knew that serious bodily harm or death would probably result from his acts. Death resulting from the commission of felony also constitutes murder.

A chiropractor was convicted of murder in the death of an 8-year-old patient. The court reversed the judgment due to prejudicial erroneous instructions to the jury. There was evidence that removal of a cancerous eye was necessary to save the child's life, but the chiropractor, with reckless and wanton cupidity, falsely represented himself to the parents as being able to cure cancer. He induced the parents to forego the operation and submit the child to his treatment. Thus, the child's life was shortened; the elements of first degree murder were present. However, the evidence could also have been weighed and accepted as showing second degree murder or manslaughter. The felony murder rule was prejudicially erroneous as binding the jury by conclusive presumption if they found the felony of theft by false pretense.[17]

First or Second Degree Murder

From reading and conversation, a nurse has heard such terms as first degree murder, second degree murder and manslaughter. Usually the distinction is not clear to her. In some states, the crime of murder is divided into first degree murder, which generally means malice aforethought plus premeditation and deliberation, and second degree murder, which is killing without premeditation or deliberation.[18] In other states, there is no distinction between first and second degree murder.

Manslaughter

By way of distinction, manslaughter means an unlawful killing of a human being without malice aforethought.[19] For example, the killing may take place during a sudden quarrel or may occur unintentionally while the person is doing some unlawful or lawful act. If the manslaughter is the result of an intentional killing without malice, it is called "voluntary"; but when the manslaughter is the result of an act without malice, and is an unintentional killing, it is called "involuntary." By way of illustration, death resulting from a person's negligently leaving poison where it may endanger life was held to be involuntary manslaughter;[20] similarly, a death due to reckless driving is usually held to be involuntary manslaughter.[21]

A case most frequently mentioned in this connection occurred over 25 years ago. In this case, a surgeon ordered the head nurse to prepare, as an anesthetic, a 10 per cent cocaine solution with Adrenalin for a tonsillectomy patient; the nurse repeated the order. After the injection, the patient convulsed and died. The doctor meant procaine in the order instead of cocaine. Here was a situation in which the nurse should have questioned the order. By reason of her training, education and experience, she should have recognized that the order was incorrect. Not only was the nurse negligent, but her conduct amounted to gross negligence. The nurse was convicted of manslaughter.[22] The lesson of this case should be thoroughly understood by all nurses.

Concerning this case, students frequently inquire why the nurse was convicted instead of the doctor. The answer is that the negligent act of the nurse caused the patient's death. The surgeon was also negligent, but his negligence in itself did not cause the death. In all likelihood, the case would not have arisen had the head nurse been alert and said, for example, "Pardon me, Doctor, did you say 10 per cent procaine?" It bears repetition that a person is always personally answerable for his own torts and negligent acts. The negligent act in this case reached the level of crime. Failure to consider causes and effects which careful nurses ought to know and to recognize gives rise to liability.

Nurses take courses in pharmacology, pharmacodynamics, anatomy, physiology, and other subjects and therefore are required to have a knowledge of cause and effect in executing orders. On occasion, though seldom, physicians have made errors in ordering medicines. The well-trained, alert, thinking nurse will tactfully check any obvious discrepancy. With a knowledge of the average therapeutic dose, the maximum dose, the effects of the drug, and the age, sex and condition of the patient, the nurse's action if there is an apparent discrepancy in an order would have to be judged by what the average, reasonable and prudent nurse would do in such circumstances.

PRINCIPALS IN FELONIES

Attention is directed at this point to the persons concerned in the commission of felonies. They are either principals or accessories.[23] In misdemeanors and in treason the distinction between principals and accessories is not recognized. A person who actually does or performs the act either himself or by an innocent agent is a principal in the first degree.[24] A person who is either actually or constructively present, aiding and abetting (encouraging, supporting) another in the commission of an act, is a principal in the second degree.[25] As between the principals, there must be a common interest of unlawful purpose at the time the act is done. To illustrate, a person who mixed paris green and water in a cup and placed it within reach of another person, who drank it and committed suicide, aided and abetted the killing and was guilty of murder.[26] A female friend who simply accompanies a woman who undergoes an illegal abortion is not an associate in guilt.[27] But if a person, say, loaned her home to a woman so that she could have an illegal abortion done therein, the person would be a party to the crime.*

---

*In the District of Columbia, the woman who has an abortion performed on herself is not an accomplice.

ACCESSORIES TO THE CRIME

A person who was absent when the act was done, but who obtained, advised, ordered, or encouraged the principal to commit it, is an "accessory before the fact."[28] A person who for the purpose of defeating justice receives, comforts, assists, or relieves another person and, at the time he does so, knows that the other person has committed a felony, is an "accessory after the fact."[29] It is pertinent to note that a person who removes evidence after a crime is an accessory after the fact. To illustrate, if a woman tells her paramour she is "in trouble" and asks his help, and he gives her a piece of paper on which is written the name and address of a person who performs illegal abortions, and if in addition he gives her the exact amount of money to pay such a person, then the paramour, although not present at the illegal abortion on the woman, may be considered an accessory before the fact. As another example, a person who helps another to dispose of a large quantity of gems, which he knows to be stolen goods, is an accessory after the fact. In most jurisdictions, a parent or spouse is immune from prosecution as an accessory after the fact. To be punishable as an accessory to a criminal act, assistance or participation must be shown.

ABORTIONS

Inasmuch as nurses may encounter problems involving abortions among their patients, this topic warrants more detailed consideration. At common law, any person who, with the intention of prematurely ending a pregnancy, willfully and unlawfully does any act which causes a miscarriage, is guilty of the crime of procuring an abortion. Today a similar wording is used in statutes defining the crime of abortion. In most of these statutes, there is a specific exemption of those abortions performed in good faith for the purpose of preserving the life of the mother. Such an abortion is commonly referred to as a therapeutic abortion. It has been said that there is a presumption that the physician acts in good faith.[30] In a widely discussed English case, a prominent English physician was tried on an abortion charge when he induced an abortion on a 15-year-old girl who had been raped.[31] The physician was acquitted. The judge said:

> There remain three further cases in which the arguments in favour of procuring abortion might be very strong. These are:
> (a) where the woman is pregnant as the result of rape;
> (b) where the woman is insane and becomes pregnant while insane;
> (c) where the woman is under the age of consent.

Recently, some states have changed their abortion laws[31a] and other states are contemplating changes.

Viewpoint of the Roman Catholic Church

On this topic, it is important to know the point of view of the Roman Catholic Curch:* In all pregnancies it is forbidden to kill the mother in order to save the child, or to kill the child in order to save the mother. However, providing a physician does what he can to save both lives, the indirect loss of one life resulting from an attempt to save the other is morally justifiable.[32]

After a criminal abortion, if a woman dies and if it can be proved that the person responsible knew that the act was likely to cause serious bodily harm or death, he can be charged with murder. When the responsible person does the act without such knowledge, he is charged with manslaughter. A wrongful unsuccessful effort to secure an abortion is called "attempting to procure an abortion," which is a crime. By statute, anyone who aids, advises, prescribes, abets or administers a drug to induce abortion in a woman, unless it is necessary to preserve her life, is criminally liable.

CRIMINAL OR GROSS NEGLIGENCE

As has been pointed out, criminal negligence or gross negligence is a commission or omission of an act, lawfully or unlawfully, in which such a degree of negligence exists as may cause a serious wrong to another. To illustrate, a paying patient in a charitable hospital, through the negligence of a nurse, was given a medicine that in fact had been intended for another patient in an adjoining room. The medicine proximately caused serious injury to the plaintiff, including the death of her baby. In a civil action for damages against the hospital, a judgment for the defendant was affirmed, since it was immune from liability as a charitable institution.[33] Nevertheless, the negligence of the nurse in question is readily apparent.

In another case in which a mother died after childbirth, a judgment for damages against a private hospital was affirmed, since there was sufficient evidence to sustain a finding that a nurse was negligent in failing to observe postpartum eclampsia and in not notifying the attending physician.[34]

In another case, a physician ordered a nurse to give a sitz bath to a patient. The nurse prepared the bath negligently, and as a result the patient was severely scalded.[35] Though the case does not state whether the nurse was a student nurse, a practical nurse or a graduate nurse, the finding of negligence on the part of the nurse would have been the same. Ordinary persons are presumed to know the dangers of excessively hot water in giving baths, and failure to

---

*Canon 2350 states: "Those who procure abortion, not excepting the mother, incur, if the effect is produced, an excommunication latae sententiae reserved to the Ordinary; and if they be clerics they are moreover to be deposed."

act in accordance with such common knowledge, when others are injured as a result, constitutes criminal negligence. In this case, since the action was brought against two doctors in the hospital rather than the negligent nurse, the verdict was for the defendant.

FRAUD

An osteopathic physician and his assistant were convicted of 22 counts of submitting false and fraudulent claims to the Bureau of Public Assistance of Los Angeles County for treatment of public welfare patients and of conspiracy to submit such claims. The conviction was reversed when the court held that admission of his private medical records, taken under a search warrant, to prove that the doctor had presented false claims for treatment of public welfare patients and had conspired to present false claims, violated the physician's constitutional privilege against self-incrimination and his privilege against unreasonable search and seizure.[36]

ASSAULT AND BATTERY

In criminal law, an assault is an attempt or offer, with force or violence, to inflict a physical injury upon another. It must consist of an actual overt (apparent) act; words are not enough.[37] There is a split of authority in the cases, but it would seem that a general criminal intent is enough. Battery is an assault in which any force, however slight, is actually applied to another. A general criminal intent is sufficient for the crime.[38]

In a New York case, the administratrix recovered damages in a civil suit for the death of her husband, whose death was from:

> . . . intra-abdominal hemorrhage, shock, and fractured ribs caused by external violence.

The patient had been suffering from dementia praecox, paranoid type, and died as result of negligence of the attendants of the Hudson River State Hospital at Poughkeepsie. The court said the attendant violated rules and regulations of his department and:

> . . . visited entirely unnecessary force toward, if not actually venting personal animosity toward a patient, while ample means were available to him of suppressing the patient however strenuous his resistance might have been.

In this case, it was brought out that the attendant had a record of conviction for:

> . . . crime of willfully inflicting harsh, cruel and unkind treatment and neglect of duty toward an incompetent person. . . .[39]

This unpleasant case illustrates a type of assault and battery.

ROBBERY

Robbery is a felony at common law, and it is a crime against the person and property. The taking of personal property of another person from him or in his presence, by either violence or intimidation and against his will, constitutes robbery.[40] Larceny at common law is obtaining personal property of another by trespass in taking and carrying away of it together with a felonious intent to deprive the person of ownership.[41]

In a Massachusetts case, a civil action was brought against a private hospital for loss of a ring while the plaintiff was undergoing an operation. There was evidence that plaintiff had engaged accommodations at the hospital for her operation and had also contracted for nursing before, after and during the operation. Furthermore, there was evidence that one of the operating room nurses stole a ring from the plaintiff's hand while she was under the influence of ether. It was held that there was a violation by the hospital of its duty toward the plaintiff under its contract with her, and that the plaintiff could sue only for breach of defendant's contractual duty.[42] The wrongdoing of the nurse was obvious, although the case was one for civil damages.

MAYHEM

Mayhem was a crime at common law which was the same as "maim," and it involved a violent injury to another, rendering him less able to fight, to annoy his enemy or to defend himself.[43] In most jurisdictions of the United States, it is a felony. For example, when a stepfather scalded a boy's feet, and the skin came off the toes so that, except for medical treatment, they would have grown together, it was held to be mayhem.[44]

RAPE

The act of having unlawful carnal knowledge of a woman by force and against her will is rape.[45] It has been held that when there is the slightest penetration, the crime is committed. The force may be either actual or constructive, as when it is induced by fear or intimidation.

POSSESSION OF NARCOTICS

A nurse should realize that, except in situations specifically exempted, both the Federal and state laws make possession of narcotics a crime. A discussion of narcotics is important because the nurse frequently administers them in her work, and she should be informed about the legal regulations in regard to them. The chief Federal narcotic laws are the Narcotic Drugs Import and Export Act,[46] the Harrison Narcotic Law;[47] the Marihuana Tax Act[48] and the Narcotics Manufacturing Act of 1960.[49] The Uniform State Narcotic Act has been adopted in 42 states. The narcotics covered by such laws include opium, coca leaves and any compound, salt or derivative or preparation of them, and isonipecaine.

The law provides that a nurse may give such narcotics under the direction and supervision of a physician or dentist. It is pointed out that the word "nurse" is used in the law, and there is no apparent distinction in the law between registered professional nurses and practical nurses regarding the administration of narcotics. Moreover, the law specifically provides that when a nurse has procured narcotics from a physician, if the same is no longer needed by the patient, the unused part is to be returned to the physician.

The nurse should appreciate that a physician or dentist is required to obtain a license to practice medicine or dentistry. In regard to nurses, the Harrison Narcotic Law provides that nurses are regarded as agents of the practitioners or institutions under whose direction and supervision their duties are performed. Therefore, under the law, a nurse may give narcotics only under the direction of a physician or dentist who is duly licensed to dispense narcotics under the Narcotic Law. Attempts to obtain narcotics by fraud or deceit are unlawful. Any violation or failure to comply with the Harrison Narcotic Law is a crime punishable by fine or imprisonment, or both. Any violation or failure to comply under the model law when it has received state adoption is a felony or high misdemeanor and is likewise punishable by fine or imprisonment, or both. Obviously, nurses should be circumspect in their habits, in handling narcotics, and in faithfully maintaining records evidencing the same.

A violation of the Harrison Narcotic Law in Arizona has been held to be an offense involving moral turpitude within the statutory definition of unlicensed professional conduct. For the violation, the person's license to practice medicine was revoked.[50] It would seem that similar conduct on the part of a nurse would bring an equivalent penalty.

There are certain practical rules that the nurse who administers narcotics should know. Any P.R.N. order for a narcotic drug must be rewritten every 72 hours. A standing order, meaning a drug dose administered for the physician by a nurse without first obtaining a signed order for each hospital patient, is not permitted for narcotic drugs. In an emergency, a verbal order for narcotic drugs is permitted if the nurse makes note of the nature of the emergency in the chart and the physician validates the order within 24 hours.

When a dose of a narcotic is refused by the patient, then in the presence of a witness, it should be placed in the sewage system. If a dose of a narcotic drug is contaminated or wasted, the nurse should make an entry in the record explaining how the dose was disposed of and it should be signed by a witness.

ADMINISTRATION OF ANESTHESIA BY NURSES

The right of a properly trained nurse to administer anesthesia is no longer a legal question. The practice of medicine involves three things: judging the nature of a disease or injury by its signs and symptoms, deciding upon the proper remedy, and prescribing it. The nurse who administers a prescribed anesthetic to a patient in the presence of and in accordance with a surgeon's directions is held not to practice medicine.[51] The attorney generals of New York,[52] Iowa,[53] South Dakota,[54] and other states have stated that administration of anesthesia by a registered nurse under the direction of a licensed physician is the practice of nursing and not medicine. Questions relative to nurse anesthetists administering endotracheal and spinal anesthesia go to the adequacy of their training, since there is no legal provision that distinguishes these from other types of anesthesia.[55]

The nurse anesthetist, like other nurses, is responsible for her own acts. Her acts are also the responsibility of her employer under the master-servant relationship.[56] If the nurse is a hospital employee, her acts while she administers anesthesia are charged to the surgeon on the borrowed servant doctrine.[57] When the act complained of arises from the use of a piece of monitoring equipment, there may be a question as to who is responsible: the manufacturer, the supplier, the hospital, the owner or the user; and resolving the question depends on the exact facts of the situation as well as the law of agency.[58]

ARTIFICIAL INSEMINATION

No nurse should assist the physician, whether in the hospital, doctor's office, clinic or elsewhere, in procedures which involve sterilization, artificial insemination or contraception without careful consideration of the legal, moral and religious implications.

While artificial insemination in people dates back at least to the Talmud, if recent magazine articles are to be given credence, there is increasing demand on physicians for the procedure. There is no state in the United States that by statute prohibits artificial insemination. In 1967, Oklahoma by statute authorized it and stated that a child thus produced was legitimate.[59]

The donor of semen in homologous insemination is the husband, and a child born as a consequence is legitimate. When the donor of the semen is a third party, it is heterologous insemination. In 1968, the California Supreme Court decided the legal issues of heterologous insemination. After 15 years of married life without children, both husband and wife consented to artificial insemination and signed a statement on a physician's letterhead in which they requested the procedure. The physician selected the semen and the name of the donor remained unknown to the couple. Following the artificial insemination, a boy was born to the wife and the husband was named as father on the birth certificate. Four years later they separated and divorced; the mother kept the child and asked for no support. Several years later, the mother was obliged to seek public assistance following illness, and a support order against the husband was secured. The court held that the woman's former husband was the lawful father and refused to rule that the artificial insemination was adulterous.[60] Following a divorce, a father was given the right to visit a child who resulted from the heterologous insemination of the wife to which he, the husband, had consented.[61] On the other hand, an Illinois trial court held that the wife who had received heterologous insemination with or without the husband's consent was guilty of adultery, and that such a child was illegitimate.[62]

Concerning artificial insemination, the Roman Catholic Church opposes it with one exception: a case in which only the husband's semen is used, and then merely to assist normal insemination to the extent necessary.[63]

REFUSAL OF BLOOD TRANSFUSION

When a patient refuses treatment and thus invites his own death, physicians, nurses and other health personnel are confronted by legal and moral problems. For years there was the legal maxim to the effect that any competent individual has the right to refuse treatment and thus to die, and the law does not compel him to accept available help. In recent years, the courts have made many exceptions to this rule.

Much of the problem revolves around patients who have religious convictions against blood transfusions. These patients belong to two groups: (1) believers in healing by faith who oppose all forms of customary medical therapy, including blood transfusions, and (2) Jehovah's Witnesses, who accept customary medical therapy except for blood transfusions. The widow and children of an employee were not allowed to recover benefits under the Workmen's Compensation Act when he refused a needed blood transfusion following a serious injury on the job.[64] When medical science prescribes a blood transfusion for a child, the child has a right to live, and the court will protect him and will not permit him to be deprived of life because his parents' religious views oppose blood transfusion.[65] The court has held that temporarily depriving parents of a minor child for the purpose of giving him a blood transfusion is not depriving them of religious freedom and of their parental rights.[66] A mother's custody of her children had as a condition the elimination of the need for her consent to necessary blood transfusions.[67]

The rule with respect to competent adults is less clear. The court may uphold the right of an adult patient to refuse a blood transfusion even at the risk of her life.[68] A release of liability form, signed by the patient, protects the hospital. In a case in which the patient was alert and competent while considering his decision, and no minors were involved, the court did not overrule his decision, and held that refusal of a needed transfusion was not the equivalent of suicide, which was a violation of state law.[69] However, when a patient had a massive hemorrhage from an ulcer, and the precariousness of her condition made a blood transfusion necessary, which both she and her husband refused, the court ordered a transfusion.[70] In a similar case, a Connecticut court ordered a blood transfusion for a Jehovah's Witness, who refused permission for it.[71]

A court has also ordered a life-saving operation on a comatose patient whose wife refused consent.[72]

Serum hepatitis is a risk assumed by patients who receive blood transfusions and no damages are awarded.[73]

REFERENCES

1. Perkins, Rollin M.: *Criminal Law.* Mineola, N.Y., Foundation Press, 1969, p. 12
2. Intent in statutory cases, i.e.: "willfully," United States v. Sioux City Stock Yards Co. 162 Fed. 556 (C.C.A. 1908); "knowingly," State v. Smith, 119 Tenn. 521, 105 S.W. 68 (1907)
3. McNaghten's Case, 10 Cl. & Fin. 200, 8 Eng. Rep. 718 (1843). Barnes: *A Century of the McNaghten Rules.* 8 *Camb. L.J.* 300 (1944), Perkins, pp. 858, 860
4. Keedy: Irresistable Impulse as a Defense in the Criminal Law. 100 *U. Pa. L. Rev.* 956 (1952)
5. State v. Brown, 36 Utah 46, 93 Pac. 521, 102 Pac. 641 (1909)
6. Sutton's Adm. v. Wood, 120 Ky. 23, 85 S.W. 201 (1905)
7. Bellandi v. Park Sanitarium Ass'n., 214 Cal. 472, 6 P 2d 508 (1931)
8. Underhill: *Criminal Evidence,* 4th ed. 1935, § 75 (70)
9. Perkins: *op. cit. supra.* note 1, p. 86
10. *Ibid.,* p. 626, 11
11. *United States Code* (1952 ed.) tit. 18, § 1; 4 *Federal Practice and Procedure,* Rules ed. § 1912
12. Perkins: *op. cit. supra.* note 1, p. 626. *In re* Henry, 15 Idaho 755, 99 Pac. 1054 (1909)
13. Perkins; *op. cit. supra.* note 1, pp. 28-106
14. *Ibid.,* p. 379, 1001
15. *Ibid.,* p. 1001
16. *Ibid.,* p. 48
17. People v. Phillips, 42 Cal. Reptr. 868 (1965)
18. Perkins: *op. cit. supra.* note 1, p. 89
19. *Ibid.,* p. 51, 96
20. Rex v. Grout, 6 Car. & P. 629, 172 Eng. Rep. 1394 (1834)
21. Lee v. State, 1 Cold 62, 41 Tenn. 42 (1860)

22. Somera Case, G.R. 31693 (Philippines Is. 1929). Grennan, Elizabeth M.: The Somera Case. *International Nursing Review,* 5:325-34, (1930)*

23. Perkins: *op. cit. supra.* note 1, pp. 623, 643, 667

24. *Ibid.,* p. 656

25. *Ibid.,* p. 657

26. People v. Roberts, 211 Mich. 187, 178 N.W. 690 (1920)

27. People v. McGonegal, 136 N.Y. 62, 32 N.E. 616 (1892)

28. Perkins: *op. cit. supra.* note 1, p. 663

29. *Ibid.,* p. 667

30. State v. Shoemaker, 157 Iowa 176, 138 N.W. 381 (1912)

31. Rex v. Bourne, 3 All E.R. 615, 186 L.T. 87 (1938), [1939] 1 K.B. 687; *Brit. Med. J.,* 1938, 2, 199; 6 *Univ. Chi. L. Rev.* 107 (1939)

31a. Foster, John F.: Abortion – Three States Have New Laws and More Are Coming. *Mod. Hosp.,* 109:90-4, Aug., 1967

32. Kelly, Gerald, S.J.: Therapeutic Abortion. *Hospital Progress,* 31:342, Nov., 1950; 370 (Dec., 1950). See also O'Donnell, Thomas J., S.J.: *Morals in Medicine.* Newman Press, Westminster, Md., 1956, p. 121 ff.

33. Enell *et al.* v. Baptist Hospital, 45 S.W. 2d 395 (Tex. Ct. of Appeals, 1931); *Hospitals,* XIII, 107 (Aug., 1939)

34. Hansch v. Hackett, 190 Wash. 97, 66 P 2d 1129 (1937). See also Valentin v. La Société Française de Bienfaisance Mutuelle, 76 Cal. App. 2d 1, 172 P 2d 359 (1946)

35. Perinowsky v. Freeman, 4 F & F. 977, 176 Eng. Rep. 873 (1866)

36. People v. Thayer, 44 Cal. Rept. 718 (1965)

37. Perkins; *op. cit. supra.* note 1, p. 132

38. *Ibid.,* p. 115-116

39. St. Pierre v. State, 33 N.Y.S. 2d 151 (Ct. Cl. 1942)

40. Perkins; *op. cit. supra.* note 1, pp. 190, 281

41. *Ibid.,* p. 234

42. Vannah v. Hart Private Hospital, 228 Mass. 132, 117 N.E. 328, L.R.A., 191 A 1157 (1917)

43. Perkins: *op. cit. supra.* note 1, p. 185, 187

44. State v. McDonie, 89 W. Va. 185, 109 S.E. 710 (1921)

45. Perkins: *op. cit. supra.* note 1, p. 152. See also Rape or Suspected Rape Cases. *J. of La. Med. Soc.,* 119: 319-320, Aug., 1967.

46. *U.S. Code* (1952 ed.), tit. 21, § 171-85; Feb. 9, 1909 c. 100 § 9; May 26, 1922, c. 202, § 4, 42 Stat. 598

47. *U.S. Code* (1952 ed.) tit. 26, § 4701-4762, Dec. 17, 1914, c. 1, 38 Stat. 785

48. 26 U.S.C. § 4741-4742 and 7237

49. 26 U.S.C. § 4731

50. Garlington v. Smith, 63 Ariz. 460, 163 P. 2d 685 (1945)

51. Frank v. Smith, 194 S.W. 375 (Ky. 1917). See also Chalmers-Francis v. Nelson, 57 P. 2d 1312 (Cal. 1936). Hayt, Emanuel: The Law and the Practice of Anesthesia. *J. Am. A. Nurse Anesthetists,* 32:373-9, Dec., 1964

52. Op. Atty. Gen. of N.Y. Nov. 15, 1933

53. Rep. of Atty. Gen. of Iowa on Registered Nurses: Administration of Anesthetics, June 27, 1946.

54. Op. Atty. Gen. of South Dakota, June 3, 1964

55. Op. Atty. Gen. of N.Y., Sept. 3, 1957

56. Prosser, W. L.: *Handbook of the Law of Torts,* 3rd ed. West, St. Paul, 1964, p. 470. Mecham, F. R.: *Outlines of the Law of Agency.* 4th ed. Callaghan and Co., Chicago, 1952, p. 327. Wasmuth, C. E.: *Anesthesia and the Law.* Charles C Thomas, Springfield, Ill., 1961, p. 33

57. Wasmuth: *op. cit. supra.* note 6, p. 41

58. Dornette, William, H. L.: Monitoring the Anesthetized Patient: Practical Aspects and Legal Connotations. *J. Am. A. Nurse Anesthetists,* 36:420-425, Dec., 1968

---

*Unfortunately, the case was not reported either in the *Official Gazette* or in the *Philippine Reports.* Miss Daisy C. Bridges, Executive Secretary of the International Council of Nurses in 1956, and Miss Julita V. Sotejo, Dean of the College of Nursing, University of the Philippines, kindly cooperated with me in endeavoring to locate all possible source material on this case.

59. *Oklahoma Annotated Laws.* Title 10 § 551-553, 1967
60. People v. Sorensen, 66 Cal. Rptr. 7, 437 P. 2d 495 (1968)
61. Strnad v. Strnad, 190 Misc. 786, 78 N.Y.S. 2d 390 (1948)
62. Doornbos v. Doornboos, 12 Ill App. 2d 473, 139 N.E. 2d 844 (1956)
63. *Linacre Quarterly,* p. 1 ff., Oct., 1949
64. Martin v. Industrial Accident Co., 304 P. 2d 828 (Cal., 1957)
65. Battaglia v. Battaglia, 172 N.Y.S. 2d 361 (1958). See also State v. Perricone, 37 N.J. 463 (1962) in which the court gave the superintendent of a hospital the custody of a child whose parents refused a blood transfusion; and Morrison v. State, 252 S.W. 2d 97 (Mo., 1952) to the same effect
66. People *ex rel.* Wallace v. Lawrenz, 104 N.E. 2d 769 (Ill., 1958)
67. Levitsky v. Levitsky, 190 A. 2d 601 (Md., 1963)
68. Brooks Estate v. Brooks, 205 N.E. 2d 435 (Ill., 1965)
69. Erickson v. Dilgard, 252 N.Y.S. 2d 705 (1962)
70. Jessie E. Jones v. President and Directors of Georgetown College, Inc., 331 Fed. 2d 1000 (1964)
71. United States v. George, 33LW2518 (Conn. 1965)
72. Collins v. Davis, 254 N.Y.S. 2d 666 (1964)
73. Sloneker v. St. Joseph's Hospital, 233 F. Supp. 105 (Colo., 1964)

Additional References

Affleck, W. B.: Coroners' Inquests. *Crim. L.Q.,* 7:459 ff., Feb., 1965
Allen, D. L.: Coverage Problems in Libel, Slander and Assault and Battery Cases. *A.B.A. Sect. Ins. N. Cl.,* p. 531 ff., 1968
Francis, J. J., *et al.:* Law, Morality and Abortion: A Symposium. *Rutgers Law Rev.* 22:415 ff., Spring, 1968
Goetsch, Carl: Aspects of Refusal of Blood Transfusion. *Am. J. Obs. & Gyn.,* 101:390-6, June, 1968
Hanson, A. B.: Developments in the Law of Libel: Impact of the *New York Times* Rule. *William and Mary Law Rev.,* 7:215 ff., May, 1966
Kabat, Hugh F.: Narcotic Laws in Relation to Geriatric Nursing. *Geriatric Nursing,* 3:10-15, Nov., 1967
Lucas, R.: Federal Constitutional Limitations on the Enforcement of State Abortion Statutes. *North Carolina Law Rev.* 46:739 ff., June, 1968
Medical, Moral and Legal Implications of Recent Medical Advances—A Symposium. Introduction (D. W. Dowd); A Perspective for Considering the Moral, Legal and Ethical Problems Arising from Advances in Medical Science (W. Likoff); The Dying Patient, the Doctor and the Law (J. R. Elkington); The Legal Problems of Organ Transplantation (E. Z. Berman); Between Life and Death; Ethical and Moral Issues Involved in Recent Medical Advances (T. A. Wassmer); The Paradoxical Preservation Principle (R. H. Potter, Jr.). *Villanova L. Rev.* 13:732 ff., Summer, 1968
Negligence—Medical Malpractice—The Locality Rule. *De Paul L. Rev.* 18:328 ff., Autumn, 1968
Prosser, W. L.: More Libel for Quod. *Harv. L. Rev.* 79:26 ff., Jan., 1966
Schechter, David C.: Problems Relevant to Major Surgical Operations in Jehovah's Witnesses. *Am. J. Surg.,* 116:73-80, July, 1968
Schreiner, G. E.: Liability: Use of Investigational Drugs. *Chicago Bar Record,* 46:234 ff., Feb., 1965

Chapter Ten

Witnesses, Dying Declarations, Wills, and Gifts

The average nurse is often unmindful of the fact that her profession makes her liable at times to be called upon to testify in regard to some matter in a legal proceeding. In general, the nurse should realize that a witness is required to testify to facts; the jury and the court must form an opinion of their own and they are not interested in the witnesses' opinions on the matters in dispute. If the problem is one which requires special study or experience to form a sound opinion, then the opinion of an expert witness who has such special experience or study is pertinent and admissible. As we have previously pointed out, no witness is required to appear and testify, nor liable to penalty for failure to do so, unless a subpoena is served on him, summoning him to court on a certain day to give evidence. If, for reasons beyond his control, a witness is unable to respond to the subpoena, he should take steps to notify the court as quickly as possible. For attendance at court, witnesses are paid a fee.

DUTIES OF A WITNESS

A witness, before giving evidence, is required to swear or solemnly affirm that he will tell the truth, the whole truth, and nothing but the truth. If, after taking an oath, a witness makes a statement which is false or which he does not know or believe to be true, then he is guilty of perjury, which is a crime. Provided that a person acts reasonably, a witness is protected from a civil action for damages when he makes a defamatory statement in evidence. In general, a witness cannot be required to answer any question if his answer would subject him to criminal prosecution. He is privileged not to answer the question. This is known as the privilege against self-incrimination. Although it is the duty of the judge to tell the witness that he does not have to answer such a question, still, the witness is reminded to be alert and to protest any such question and ask whether he must answer it. Since a person is allowed to attack the credibility of his opponent's witness, a nurse can appreciate how the problem arises as to whether a particular question is privileged on the ground of incriminating the witness or is a legitimate question to attack the credit which might be given to the witness's evidence.

A witness is under a duty to do all that he can to assist the course of justice. The nurse is reminded that unless a person is impartial, this matter of assisting justice is well-nigh impossible. She knows only too well the human tendency to see and to hear only that which a person wants to see and to hear. The oath of a witness, as noted, requires that she tell the truth, the whole truth, and nothing but the truth.

The witness should speak loudly enough to be readily heard. The witness should give a simple, direct answer to the question asked and no more. Loquacious, chatty answers not only consume the valuable time of the court, but also often form a basis for a protracted, difficult cross-examination. Again, the nurse should be reminded to use words and terms that the average person will understand. For example, the witness might tell a juror that on May 25 the skin around the plaintiff's right eye was tumefied and contused, or she might relate that on May 25 the plaintiff had a black eye. Suffice it to say that the ordinary, reasonable man knows what you mean by a black eye.

LAW OF EVIDENCE

After this brief discussion of witnesses, a few words about evidence are in order. Several volumes would be needed for any detailed discussion of the law of evidence, but a few points may help the nurse's understanding of this important phase of law.

Tangible Evidence

Evidence is any type of proof legally presented at the trial of an issue by the act of the parties and through the medium of witnesses, documents, concrete objects, records, and so forth, for the purpose of persuading the jury or court as to their contention.[1] In a legal case, evidence is admissible when it is of such a kind that the court is obliged to receive it. The court, for example, will take judicial notice of facts and matters of common and general knowledge, such as that aspirin and citrate of magnesia are drugs.[2]

Another kind of evidence is the testimony of witnesses. For example, testimony that the adjustment of splints and bandages upon a plaintiff's injured arm was so tight that there was no allowance of space for swelling was admissible evidence.[3] However, in this connection it is pointed out that a statement of a person which is of a self-serving nature is not admissible as evidence in his favor.[4] Nor may a witness bring in evidence which is irrelevant or immaterial to the issues (matters in dispute) of the case. The judge or jury (if it is a trial by jury) decides on the weight to be given testimony of witnesses and the witnesses' credibility. Statements against interest are admissible. A witness may refresh her memory by looking over records or charts made by her at a time when the facts were fresh in her mind. If a nurse is a witness, she cannot read statements from nursing books to a jury. Witnesses may exhibit other material things to the senses. For example, in a Maryland case, a plaintiff was allowed to show her injured knees to the jury.[5]

"Hearsay" Evidence

Perhaps the nurse has heard of "hearsay evidence." When a witness gives testimony which is simply a repetition of what he has heard others say, it is called hearsay evidence and is not admissible. For instance, when a plaintiff gave testimony as to what a nurse who had helped at an operation on the plaintiff later told her about the way the operation was done, the testimony was not admissible.[6] In other words, in that case the plaintiff was not testifying from her personal knowledge, but simply repeating what she had heard another say; hence it was hearsay evidence and not admissible.

Truth Serum and Lie Detector Tests

In reply to the frequent inquiry of nurses about truth serum tests and lie detector tests as evidence of a person's guilt in connection with a crime, the courts usually reject such tests.[7] However, evidence of a urinalysis test for alcohol is admissible in many jurisdictions.

DYING DECLARATIONS

Perhaps a few words about dying declarations may be instructive to a nurse. A statement concerning the cause of his injury or illness made by a person who believes he is dying and has no hope of recovery is a dying declaration. Generally, dying declarations may be admitted in cases of murder or a felonious homicide. For example, the court allowed a defendant to show the dying declaration of the dead person when the defendant was being prosecuted for the killing of the deceased.[8] A dying delcaration may be verbal, but the nurse or person receiving it should put it in writing either while it is being made or as soon afterward as she can. The person's actual words should be written down if possible. When it can be done, the dying declaration should be read back to the person to see whether it is correct. If possible, the person making the dying declaration should sign the statement and persons present should witness the signature.

WILLS

The topic of statements made by dying persons leads to statements of a testamentary (pertaining to a will) character. On the following pages, who may make a will and the elements of testamentary capacity are discussed. Wills which are made orally are called nuncupative wills. As a well-known authority on wills has stated, the statutes of most states with certain restrictions recognize an oral will for disposing of personal property as valid.[9] Common restrictions are that the will be made during the person's last illness, that it be done in the place in which he died, that he asked one or more of the required witnesses to witness the will, that the matter of the will be put in writing within a given number of days, that the will be offered for probate (official proof) within a specified time, and that the amount of property passing by an oral will is generally limited.[10] A nuncupative will dictated by a person in his last illness before the required number of witnesses and later recorded is valid.[11]

Law Regarding Wills

A brief review of the law regarding wills may be of interest to the nurse. The nurse is not trained in the techniques or law of executing a will. Therefore, the nurse should not offer to perform this service for another person. When a patient asks a nurse for such help, the best thing she can do is to advise him to consult an attorney. A nurse has no more right to engage in the practice of law than she has to engage in the practice of medicine. However, since nurses frequently care for patients who are near death, when there is no time to consult an attorney, a nurse may assist the patient with a will. It is to help a nurse in such "emergency" situations that a limited amount of material on the topic is offered.

A will is a declaration of a person's mind as to what is to be done after his death with his property. A will may be revoked during his lifetime. It is operative for no purpose until his death, and it applies to the situation as it exists at his death.[12]

Disposal of property. In connection with wills, the nurse is likely to encounter a number of new terms such as "real property" and "personal property." Real property is land and generally whatever is erected on, or growing upon, or fastened to land.[13] Often, in a general way, real property is therefore regarded as "immovables." Personal property is everything that is owned that does not come under the denomination of real estate. Again, personal property is sometimes spoken of as "movables." Under personal property, a nurse may hear of "corporeal" personal property, which includes movable and tangible things such as furniture, animals and merchandise; and "incorporeal" personal property, which consists of such items as stocks, patents and copyrights.[14] A person is said to "bequeath" personal property by will, whereas a person is said to "devise" real property.

Factors necessary for a valid will. A person must have testamentary capacity to make a valid will, and testamentary capacity to make a will is determined according to a person's mental ability to make a will.

SOUND MIND. To execute a valid will, one must be of "sound mind"; however, a person does not have to have an above-average mind intellectually or even average mentality.[15] For the purpose of making a will, a person has a sound mind only when he can understand and carry in his mind in a general way the following: the type and amount of his property, the persons who are the natural objects of his generosity and their claims on him, and the disposition he is making of his property.[15] In addition, he must be able to appreciate such factors in relation to each other and to make an orderly desire as to the disposition of his property.[16] If a person lacks the above qualifications, then he is not mentally competent to make a will.[17] However, a person may have a guardian and may lack ability to transact some other business and yet have testamentary capacity. The nurse's attention is also invited to the fact that illiteracy, moral depravity, extreme old age, severe illness, and great weakness do not necessarily disqualify a person from making a will.[18] A person with epilepsy has been held capable of making a valid will,[19] as have a person with a brain tumor[20] and a person with apoplexy.[21] In other words, though the mental power may be reduced below the ordinary standard, yet if there is enough intelligence to understand the act of making a will in the different aspects already mentioned, there is capacity to make a will.[22]

FREEDOM FROM FRAUD AND UNDUE INFLUENCE. It is also necessary in order for the will to be valid that a person was free from the effect of fraud and undue influence when he made the will. Obviously, when a patient is in a weakened condition, it might be possible for a person particularly close to him to induce the patient to make him a beneficiary in the will. Heirs at law or beneficiaries under earlier wills of the deceased, or in general anyone who will be directly benefited by setting aside a will, may contest it.[23] Frequently, relatives of the deceased and others who think that they should have benefited by the will, or those who have been named and think they have been treated unfairly, take the matter to court.

LEGAL AGE REQUIREMENT.   In many states, minors, unless they are married, are not considered competent to make a will.

Intestacy.   A person who dies without a will is said to die intestate. His personal property and the real property of a person who made a nuncupative will are distributed according to the law of intestacy.

Execution of a will.   Statutes govern the formalities[24] for the execution of a will. Ordinarily, a will must be in writing. Nuncupative wills, for obvious reasons, tend to be frowned upon by courts. A will must be signed; however, a mark is sufficient (it would have to be properly identified by one who could write). A person does not have to write his full name. In most states, two competent witnesses are required to sign the will, whereas a few states require three witnesses. If more than the required number of witnesses sign a will, the will is not made invalid by their so doing. The person making the will should sign the will before the witnesses subscribe; a few states require signing by the person making the will, in the presence of the witnesses to it. In some states, statutes expressly require that a person making a will request the witnesses to act as witnesses. In the absence of an express statutory provision, it is usually not required that the person making the will publish (tell the witnesses) that the document is his will. The witnesses must sign the document with the intention of giving validity to such a document as the act of the person making the will.

The nurse should know that it is practically a universal requirement in the statutes that the witnesses should all be present at the same time and should sign the will in the presence of the person making the will. For example, if a blind person is making a will, then he and his witnesses should all be present at the same time. He would sign his will, and the witnesses would sign it "in his presence," which is sufficient, although the blind person cannot actually "see" the witnesses do it. Witnesses to a will should not be beneficiaries under the will, because in most jurisdictions it does affect their right to take under the will if there are not a sufficient number of witnesses who do not stand to benefit by the will.

For the protection of the nurse, she should make a notation on the patient's chart of the apparent mental and physical condition of the patient at the time of making the will and also the fact of his making the will. Such records may be important if the will is later contested.

Example of a Will

The following example will illustrate the formalities for the execution of a will:[25]

Last will and testament of_____. I,_____, of (or "residing in") the city (or as the case may be) of_____, county of_____, state of_____, being of sound mind and disposing mind and memory, and not acting under duress, menace, fraud or undue influence of any person whomsoever, do make, publish and declare this my last will and testament, and I do hereby expressly revoke all other and former wills and codicils to wills made by me.

First. I direct my executors hereinafter named to pay all my just debts and obligations, including the expenses of my last sickness, as soon after my decease as is practicable.

Second. I bequeath the following property to the persons hereinafter named.

    1. To_____, my_____automobile.

    2. To_____, my household furniture consisting of_____.

    3. To_____,

Third. I bequeath the following sums of money to the persons and associations hereinafter named:

    1. To_____, _____dollars.

    2. To_____, _____dollars.

Fourth. I devise the following real property to the persons hereinafter named:

    1. To my wife,_____(name), _____(describe property).

    2. To my son,_____(name), _____(describe property).

    3. To my daughter,_____(name), _____(describe property).

Fifth. (If any property devised or bequeathed in trust) I devise and bequeath to_____(or "_____and_____" or the like)_____(describe property) in trust, however, for the following purposes, viz.,_____.

Sixth. (If there is a trust) the trustees shall be bound to observe the following instructions in handling the property devised and bequeathed to them in trust thereby:

    1._____.

    2._____.

    3._____.

Seventh. (If a trust is included) Upon final termination of this trust, I give, bequeath and devise as follows:_____.

Eighth. All the rest and residue of my estate, of every kind and description, whether real, personal, or mixed, wherever located, I give, bequeath and devise to_____(or add: "in trust for the following purposes," etc.)

Ninth. I hereby nominate and appoint_____(or "_____and_____," or the like) to be the executor of this my last will and testament, and direct that he (or "each") be required to furnish a bond as such in the sum of_____dollars

(or direct that he [or "they"]) shall not be required to give any
bond (or "bonds") as such executor (or "executors")
Tenth. My executor (or "executors") is (or "are") hereby empowered and authorized to_____.

In witness whereof, I, (followed by the name of the testator),
have hereunto set my hand this_____ day of_____,
19_____, at the city (or as the case may be) of_____,
county_____, state of_____. Signed, sealed, published,
and declared by testator,_____, as and for his last will and
testament, in the presence of us, who, at his request, in his presence,
and in the presence of each other, have hereunto subscribed our
names as witnesses this_____day of_____, 19_____.

Insurance policies upon a person's life constitute a valid nontes-
tamentary arrangement, although the insured person retains the
right to change the beneficiary.[26]

Holographic Will

A will that is entirely written, dated and signed by the person
making the will himself is called a holographic will. By statute, in 19
states holographic wills are valid without formal attestation, that is,
without subscribing witnesses.[27]

GIFTS

However, the nurse should realize that a will is not the only way
of disposing of a person's property. Another way of disposing of a
person's property is by gift. The four legal requirements for a gift are:
the gift must consist of personal property, there must be an intention
to make the gift, an indication of transfer of control over such property, and there must be acceptance by the recipient.

The kinds of gifts with which a nurse might be especially concerned are the gifts made by dying patients. Gifts made by a person
because of approaching death or a belief in approaching death are
called gifts *causa mortis,* which are revocable and subject to the
claims of the donor's creditors without proof of intent to defraud
them.[28] Such gifts are limited to personal property. On a number of
occasions, a nurse may be asked to witness the making of such gifts
and to testify to the same. As with the execution of a will, the law
will not acknowledge the validity of a gift made by someone who does
not know what he is doing. If a patient makes the gift, he must intend
and realize the consequence of his act. Moreover, he must do it freely,
without undue influence or fraud. If a nurse doubts that a patient has
the ability to understand what he is doing, she should say so openly
and positively. Again, a nurse should make notes of the patient's
condition and reactions for the record.

In conclusion to this brief account of law that every nurse should know, I would like to call to the nurse's attention one other well-known and helpful rule of living:

> Give thought to this day, for each day well-lived, gives hope for tomorrow.

REFERENCES

1. Wigmore: 1 *Evidence,* 3rd ed. 1940, § 1. McCormick: *Handbook of the Law of Evidence.* Hornbook, 1954.
2. People v. Garcia, 1 Cal. App. 2d 761, 32 P 2d 445 (1934)
3. Klodek v. May Creek Logging Co., 71 Wash. 573, 129 Pac. 99 (1913)
4. Farmer v. Williams, 92 Vt. 132, 102 Atl. 932 (1918)
5. Zeller v. Mayson, 168 Md. 663, 179 Atl. 179 (1935)
6. Cook v. Coleman, 90 W. Va. 748, 111 S.E. 750 (1922)
7. See A.L.R. 2d 1310 for annotations and compilations of cases on this topic
8. People v. Costa, 67 Cal. App. 175, 227 Pac. 201 (1924)
9. Atkinson: *Wills.* Hornbook, 1937, § 135
10. *Ibid.,* § 135, notes 98 and 99; § 4, note 73. Bordwell: Statute Law of Wills. 14 *Iowa L. Rev.* 1, 172, 283, 428 (1928-29)
11. Starks v. Lincoln, 316 Mo. 483, 291 S.W. 132 (1927). For nuncupative wills in Louisiana, see 5 *West's Louisiana Stat. Ann.,* c. 6, § 2, art. 1574 (1952 ed. and 1955 supp.). Lemann: Testamentary Transfer Simulations. 29 *Tul. L. Rev.* 55 (1955)
12. Atkinson: *op. cit. supra.* note 9, § 1. See also *Restatement, Property,* 2d ed. 1954, § 8; and Burby: *Real Property,* 2d ed. 1954
13. 1 *Restatement, Property,* 2d ed. 1954, § 8. See also §§ 14-18; see also Moynihan: *Law of Real Property.* c. 1, 2 § 1-3 (1940)
14. 2 *Kent Comm.,* 12th ed. 1884, § 340
15. Atkinson: *op. cit. supra.* note 9, § 51
16. *In re* Whitworth's Estate, 110 Cal. App. 256, 294 Pac. 84 (1931)
17. *In re* Halbert's Will, 15 Misc. 308, 37 N.Y.S. 757 (1895)
18. Atkinson: *op. cit. supra.* note 9, § 53
19. *In re* Derusseau's Will, 175 Wis. 140, 184 N.W. 705 (1921)
20. *In re* Fricke, 64 Hun 639, 19 N.Y.S. 315 (1892)
21. Cheney v. Price, 90 Hun 238, 37 N.Y.S. 117 (1895)
22. Wood-Renton: Testamentary Capacity in Mental Disease. 4 *Law Q.R.,* 442 (1888). Green: Public Policy Underlying the Law of Mental Incompetence. 38 *Mich. L. Rev.* 1189, 1217 (1940)
23. Atkinson: *op. cit. supra.* note 9, § 99. Powell and Locker: Decedents Estates. 30 *Col. L.R.* 919 (1930)
24. Atkinson: *op. cit. supra.* note 9, § 62-72
25. 9 Nichols: *Legal Forms Annotated* (1936 ed.) 465; (1950 supp.) 441
26. Atkinson: *op. cit. supra.* note 9, § 39
27. *Ibid.,* § 75. See comprehensive note on holographic wills, 28 *Yale L.J.* 72 (1918). Parker: History of the Holographic Testament in the Civil Law. 3 *Jurist,* 1 (1943); 7 *Mont. L. Rev.* 76 (1940)
28. Atkinson: *op. cit. supra.* note 9, § 45. Mechem: Delivery in Gifts of Chattels. 21 *Ill. L. Rev.* 341, 356 (1926)

Additional References

American Jurisprudence, Vols. 56 and 57 on wills, especially §§ 217-232

Analysis of the History and Present Status of American Wills Statutes. *Ohio S. Law J.* 28:293 ff., Spring, 1967

Kerns, W. H.: The Anatomy of a Bequest. *Mod. Hosp.,* 109:112-121, Oct., 1967

Regan, William A.: It Will Pay You to Make a Will. *RN,* 28:83-90, April, 1965

Chapter Eleven

Canadian Law and Legal Practice

THE PRACTICE OF NURSING IN CANADA

The advance of the nursing profession in Canada has paralleled its growth in the United States. From the legal standpoint, both countries have sought to encourage the professionalization of nursing. It must be remembered that Canada is a federalized nation, as is the United States. There is a division of governmental authority between the central government at Ottawa and the provinces. However, there is this significant difference: In Canada, all powers not granted to the provinces are retained by Ottawa, whereas in the United States the powers not granted to the Federal government are retained by the states or the people. The power to legislate in respect to the practice of nursing in Canada is assigned to the provincial legislatures.[1]

The civil law of Quebec differs materially from the common law in the other Canadian provinces. The Quebec Civil Code, with the Code of Napoleon as a basic pattern, codifies the old French law of Quebec as modified by statutes.[2] In the United States, the civil law of Louisiana, likewise, has been influenced by the Code of Napoleon.

Examination of Provincial Nursing Acts

An examination of the various provincial nursing acts discloses the differences from province to province in regard to the licensing provisions, protection of title and practice, and causes for revocation.[3]

Development of Professionalism

As for the development of professionalization under private auspices, note must be taken of the groundwork laid by the alumnae associations of individual nursing schools. From the founding of the first of these schools at the Toronto General Hospital in 1894 to the creation of provincial associations and ultimately to membership in the International Council in 1909, Canadian nursing has acquired a status equal to that of any country.*

THE NURSE-PATIENT RELATIONSHIP

It is believed that many nurses will be interested in reading Peter Wright's article, "What Is a Profession?"[4]

Agency

The nurse and the patient may be brought together through the services of a registry. In Canada, as in the United States, there are nurses' registries. The legal relationship of the agency *vis-a-vis* the patient and the nurse is the same as that in the United States; i.e., the agency is usually regarded as the agent of the patient.[5] The liability of nurses' registries or nursing cooperations was adjudicated in *Hall v. Lees*.[6] A philanthropic association supplied nurses to patients, one of whom underwent an operation and engaged a nurse from the association to attend her in her home. The patient was burned by a hot water bottle while she was still under the anesthetic. It was held that the liability of the association depended upon the contract the patient had in fact made with the association. If the association undertook to nurse the plaintiff, it was responsible for the negligence of the nurse through whom it nursed her; if, however, it only undertook to supply a competent nurse, then its only duty to the patient was to use ordinary care and skill in selecting the nurse.

Contracts

As soon as a nurse undertakes to care for a patient, a contractual relationship is established between her and her patient. The law immediately imposes certain rights and obligations upon each of

---

*Fidler and Gray: *Law and the Practice of Nursing,* pp. 74-5: "In all Provinces except Prince Edward Island and Ontario it is necessary for a nurse to join her Provincial association in order to be registered. In seven provinces the Nursing Acts put registration under the control of the organized nursing profession, in some cases jointly with the Provincial university. In Prince Edward Island and Ontario membership in the association is voluntary, with the result that the nurses of Ontario particularly do not have anything like proportionate representation in the Canadian Nurses' Association."

them. A contract may be express or implied. An *express* contract is an actual agreement of the parties, the terms of which are openly uttered or declared at the time of making it, being stated in distinct and explicit language, either orally or in writing. An *implied* contract is one not created or evidenced by the explicit agreement of the parties, but inferred by the law from their acts or conduct. Both express and implied contracts are enforceable at law, assuming the necessary requisites are present.

Definition of contract. Contractual capacity under Canadian law requires the same elements as under American jurisprudence.[7] There must be competent parties entertaining contractual intent, an offer, an acceptance, and consideration moving from one party to the other. Liability for nursing services administered to infants, incompetents, dependent relatives and spouses follows the law in force in the United States, with a few important exceptions. For example, the Hospitals Act[8] established a new and simple principle governing the liability of a husband for hospital services provided for his wife. This liability is entirely unrelated to the law previously settled as to the husband's liability for necessities furnished his wife. The application of the new legislation was seen in *Sisters of Charity of Northwest Territories v. Ryan.*[9] The defendant husband was adjudged liable for a hospital bill incurred by his wife even though they were living apart. The plaintiff conceded that the wife had left her husband without sufficient justification and had also refused to return to him. Moreover, the wife had been receiving support which was sufficient for all her necessities, including hospital services. The court decreed that no agreement between the spouses could defeat or avoid the obligations to the hospital imposed by the Hospitals Act. In other words, absolute liability was imposed upon the husband.[10]

As noted above, when a nurse takes a case, she thereby enters into a contractual relation with the patient. More often than not, this is an oral contract, but just as binding as a written contract. The dichotomy of express and implied contracts is recognized in Canadian law.* An example of an implied contract would be the legal relationship between a nurse and an unconscious patient who is the beneficiary of her professional services. Notwithstanding that no agreement, written or oral, was entered into between the parties, the law raises up a contract and calls it an "implied contract." The case of *Hill v. Canadian National Railways*[11] is instructive in reference to the subject of implied contracts. Referring to the physician-patient-third person relationship, Justice Hope noted:

> The law does not raise an implied promise on the part of a person who requests a physician to perform services for another to

---

*For a description of these legal terms, the reader is referred to page 28, where American law and practice are discussed.

pay for the services so rendered unless the relation of such person to the patient is such as puts him under a legal obligation to provide medical attention for the patient and unless the circumstances, including the acts and conduct, are such as to show an intention on his part to pay for the services, and it is immaterial whether or not the case is one of emergency.

In summary, the nurse should remember that the mere fact that a third person has called a nurse to look after a patient is not sufficient grounds for holding the third person liable for payment of services rendered.* The parents or guardians of an infant or mentally incompetent are legally obligated to supply necessities to their child, and medical care is a necessity. A husband, as noted, must meet the medical expenses incurred by his wife.

In Quebec, nurses, physicians and dentists who fail to obtain a license to practice are precluded from recovering in a suit for services rendered. The contract with the patient in such a case is not enforceable at law.[13]

THE NURSE'S LIABILITY FOR NEGLIGENCE

Liability for negligence does not depend on a legal relationship or a contract between the nurse and the patient.† A nurse who in some manner causes injury to a patient can be sued by the patient regardless of who may have employed her or compensated her, or even whether the services were given for pay or gratuitously.

Obligations of Care and Skill Necessary

The degree of care and skill requisite to satisfy the duty which the nurse incurs in pursuing her profession was set forth in no more succinct terms than those of Chief Justice Tindal in the leading case of *Lanphter v. Phipos,* in which he charged the jury as follows:

> What you will have to say is this, whether you are satisfied that the injury sustained is attributable to the want of a reasonable and proper degree of care and skill in the defendant's treat-

---

*Nor is a person who calls a doctor to treat a patient obligated to pay for the services rendered in the absence of an agreement, express or implied, to the contrary.[12]

†*Salmond on the Law of Torts*[14] (*aliter* in other branches of law, e.g., trusts and criminal law) does not recognize different standards of care or different degrees of negligence in different classes of cases. The sole standard is the care that would be shown in the circumstances by a reasonably careful man, and the sole form of negligence is the failure to use this amount of care. It is true, indeed, that this amount will be different in different cases, for a reasonable man will not show the same anxious care when handling an umbrella as when handling a sword.[15] Again, a man may hold himself out as having a special skill which he does not in fact possess, and then the maxim *imperitia culpae adnumeratur* applies. The negligence does not consist in the lack of skill, but in undertaking the work without skill.[16]

ment. Every person who enters into a learned profession undertakes to bring to the exercise of it a reasonable degree of care and skill. He does not undertake, if he is an attorney, that at all events you shall gain your case, nor does a surgeon undertake that he will perform a cure; nor does he undertake to use the highest possible degree of skill. There may be persons who have higher education and greater advantages than he has, but he undertakes to bring a fair, reasonable, and competent degree of skill, and you will say whether, in this case, the injury was occasioned by the want of such skill in the defendant.[17]

Moreover, as under American jurisprudence, even if there be no duty on the nurse's part to do an act or take a certain precaution, she may be rendered liable if damages accrue from negligent or improper performance of such an act or precaution, even if done gratuitously.[18] As was pointed out previously, the nurse is personally liable in a civil action if a patient is injured because of carelessness in the performance of her skills and duties. Furthermore, if her negligent act reflects a wanton and reckless disregard for human life, such a degree of negligence is tantamount to "gross negligence," which the law considers criminal. However, if a surgeon intentionally performs an operation without authorization, neither the hospital nor the assisting nurse can be held liable for the negligence which occurs in the course of the operation. This result follows because the nurse is not then under the hospital's control, but is subject to the sole charge of the surgeon. Inasmuch as a nurse cannot prevent a surgeon from performing an unauthorized operation and thereby committing an assault, neither she nor the hospital is answerable therefor.[19]

It should be mentioned at this point that in an action based on negligence, a hospital record is not privileged from production, and a platintiff is entitled to make a copy of the record under statutory right.[20]

In England, it has been held that if a patient requests a doctor to give him particulars of his condition or illness to be used in a court of law, when those particulars are vital to the success or failure of the case, the doctor must comply with the request.[21] In any jurisdiction, accurate and complete records best serve the requirements of medical practice as well as justice. Furthermore, it would seem most desirable that all persons who have access to doctors' or hospitals' patients' records should be thoroughly instructed to preserve their confidential character.

Doctrine of Proximate Cause of Injury

The doctrine of proximate cause as an element in a negligence claim has also received recognition in numerous Canadian decisions. For a negligent act to be actionable, the breach of duty on the part of the nurse must be the "proximate cause of injury," that is, the injury must be one that in the usual course of events would not happen in the absence of the cause. An interesting case in which the doctrine constituted the defense was *Brandeis v. Weldon.*[22] In this case, a female patient escaped from a hospital during a short absence of the nurse in charge. On the following day, the patient's body was found drowned in a creek in the vicinity of the hospital. Her husband sought damages for negligence on the grounds that the hospital had not notified him of the patient's disappearance. On appeal, the verdict, which the plaintiff had won, was reversed; the appeal court ruled that there was no evidence from which a jury could reasonably find the physician or his nurse guilty of want of reasonable care in discharging their duties. There was nothing to show that the escape was the result of negligence on the part of the hospital staff.

The doctrine of proximate cause is applicable even when the causal agent is unknown. For example, when a patient in a hospital was burned by a hot water bottle while he was under anesthetic, the hospital was liable for the negligence of its employee, a nurse, even though none of the nurses and physicians seemed to be able to remember or account for how the hot water bottle was placed next to the patient.[23]

Legal Status of Public Health and Industrial Nurses

Before leaving the subject of the status of the nurse, mention should be made of the legal status of the public health nurse and the industrial nurse. The public health nurse is employed by an official governmental agency and is without question the most significant link in the chain of events which implement the programs set up pursuant to legislation.

> Concerning her legal status, it would appear that the public health nurse, with the exception of the industrial nurse, is not an independent contractor. If the nurse is an employee of an official agency, she is responsible administratively to the Medical Office of Health either directly or through the nursing supervisor or director.[24]

As for the industrial nurse, she should see that she is supplied with standing orders from a physician or medical association. This should be done for her own protection and that of the workers and the company by whom she is employed. As pointed out by an authority on the subject:

> The legal position of the nurse in the new field of industrial nursing is less well-defined and less secure than that of most other groups. She should therefore take special precautions to safeguard it.[25]

Liability of Hospitals for Negligence of Nurses

Canadian law recognizes various degrees of responsibility for acts negligently performed. The distinctions of employer, employee, servant and independent contractor have been recognized in statutory and case law.[26] As Salmond observed in his discussion of this aspect of the law:

> These principles have been much discussed in a series of cases dealing with the liability of hospital authorities for their staff. For many years uncertainty prevailed because of the opinion expressed in *Hillyer v. St. Bartholomew's Hospital* (1909) 2 K.B. 820, 829 per Kennedy, L.J., that a hospital was not responsible for the negligence of its professional staff (including trained nurses) in matters involving professional care and skill as distinct from matters of purely administrative nature. But in *Gold v. Essex C.C.* (1942) 2 K.B. 293 the Court of Appeal repudiated this opinion and held a hospital liable for the negligence of a radiographer employed under a full-time contract service. The position of the permanent medical staff was considered by Hilbery, J., in *Collins v. Hertfordshire C.C.*, (1947) K.B. 598 (lethal solution of cocaine injected instead of harmless procaine) where the defendants were held liable for the negligence of a resident house-surgeon employed under a contract of service, and by the (English) Court of Appeal in *Cassidy v. Ministry of Health* (1951) 2 K.B. 343. . . . It is doubtful how far the hospital is liable for the acts of its nurses done in the operating theaters on the orders of the surgeon. Gold's Case (1942) 2 K.B. 293.

So it is seen that a Canadian hospital authority is liable for the negligent acts and omissions of nurses and others in its employ, when the negligence occurs during the course of their regular duties for the hospital. The dichotomy between professional and routine acts, upon which the former leading case of Hillyer turned, has been abandoned, for all intents and purposes.* More recently, in 1952, the Supreme Court of Canada affirmed a judgment of the British Columbia Court of Appeal in holding a hospital liable for the negligence of an intern during the course of his professional duties.[27]

In 1951, a court said:

> When hospital authorities undertake to treat a patient and themselves select and appoint and employ the professional men and women who are to give the treatment, then they are responsible for the negligence of these persons in failing to give proper treatment, no matter whether they are doctors, surgeons, nurses or anyone else.[28]

It was held that the hospital undertook to treat the patient and was responsible for the negligence of its interns, and that there was

---

*This is the conclusion of Mr. Justice Doull in *Petite v. MacLeod* et al.[29] "Professional qualifications do not make the person employed any less the 'servant' of his employer if he is acting in the service of his 'master' and within the scope of his employment. A doctor or a nurse may be a 'servant' just as readily as a dishwasher."

evidence on which the jury might properly find that the death of the patient resulted from his discharge from the hospital owing to the intern's negligence either in not reading the x-ray films correctly or in not calling a radiologist. The nurse's notes and the history sheet were of some importance at the trial.[29] It should be pointed out that a hospital is not responsible for the negligence of a physician engaged and paid by the patient, even though he uses the nursing services and other facilities of the hospital.[30]

The first duty of the nurse is to carry out loyally and completely all reasonable and legal orders of the medical doctor. However, the nurse is personally liable for her wrongful acts and negligent acts. The decisions are legion in which recoveries were allowed for injuries sustained by patients and traceable to negligent acts of nurses in attendance. The doctrine of *respondeat superior* ("let the master answer") has been invoked to impress liability upon the hospital for the negligent performance of duties by a nurse employed by the hospital.[31]

Liability of charitable hospitals. An interesting suit which led to a discussion of the liability of charitable hospitals was *Beatty v. Sisters of Misericorde of Alberta.*[32] There it was said that hospitals, whether charitable institutions or otherwise, when sued for damages for negligence of their employees, are in exactly the same position as other persons, and whether or not the plaintiff can succeed depends upon the facts of the particular case.

The legal status of municipal hospitals, as far as liability for the negligence of their servants is concerned, was adjudicated in *Butler v. Toronto.*[33] In that case, the plaintiff brought action for damages for the death of his child in an isolation hospital maintained by the defendant city, under the Public Health Act.[34] Justice Clute observed:

> Even if the officers of the (municipal) board of health are paid by the corporation of the city . . . it does not follow that they are servants in such a sense that the corporation is responsible for their negligent acts.

Legal status of municipal hospitals. The basis of liability of a municipal hospital was spelled out in *Eek v. Board of High River Municipal Hospital,*[35] in which liability was imposed upon the hospital. Justice Simmons noted:

> Another test which might be applied is the control or lack of control over the nurse in attendance and the evidence quite clearly indicates that the nurse in charge was under the entire control and direction of the defendant corporation and in no way under the control and direction of the plaintiff. In the result then, I find the defendant corporation liable for negligence of an employee in regard to placing the hot water bottles at the plaintiff's feet with the result that the plaintiff has suffered injuries.

Another case involving a public hospital turned upon the fact of whether or not the nurse was acting in a professional capacity under orders of a surgeon or performing routine duty. The court held that the responsibility of the hospital is limited to securing competent professional staff and apparatus and is not liable for their professional mistakes except for acts of purely ministerial or administrative character.[36]

Liability of private hospitals. In cases involving private hospitals, whether the hospital as well as the employee is liable for damages resulting from an act of the latter depends on whether that person exercised ordinary care at the time that the injury occurred. When the nurse is acting within the scope of her duties as the servant or agent of the proprietors of a private hospital, liability falls upon the proprietors for negligent acts of the nurse.[37] A hospital which retains the services of competent medical doctors and nurses and provides proper apparatus for the treatment of patients is not responsible for the negligence of the doctors and nurses while performing their professional duties.[38]

There is no difference between professional and nonprofessional acts. The only question is whether the nurse was acting in the course of her employment as servant or agent of the hospital at the time that she was negligent. If she was so acting, the hospital would be liable for her negligence. The same principle applies to doctors. A doctor may be an employee or "servant" of a hospital, in which case the hospital is liable for his negligence within the scope of his employment, or the doctor may be operating independently — that is, he may be engaged by the patient to operate and paid by the patient, even though he makes use of the operating room and the nursing services of the hospital — in which case the hospital is not liable. As noted previously, the doctor in the latter case is liable for his own negligence.[39]

There can be negligence on the part of both the doctor and the nurse. One is a check against the other in such cases, but each has his or her own duty, which must be done with the care which a reasonable and competent person would exercise in a matter of such importance.[40]

In passing, it should be noted that visiting surgeons and physicians are not the servants of the hospital governors, and the latter are not liable for the negligence of such professional people if they have been selected with due care. Nor are the student nurses usually classed as employees. On the other hand, trained nurses, matrons, radiographers and so forth, though skilled, are the servants of the hospital, and for their negligence the hospital authorities will be liable.[41]

ILLUSTRATIONS OF NEGLIGENCE AND MALPRACTICE

The paragraphs which follow present a survey of the many types of cases involving negligence or malpractice in Canada in the field of nursing.

Negligence

Negligence has been defined as:

> ... the omission to do something which a reasonable man guided upon those considerations which ordinarily regulate the conduct of human affairs, would do, or doing something which a prudent and reasonable man would not do."[42]

Negligence is said to consist of two elements, the duty to take care and the breach of that duty.* The duty is restricted at the common law to physical injury either to the person or to property.[44] The burden of proving both elements of negligence rests upon the plaintiff at the outset of litigation.[45] The plaintiff must establish that there was a legal duty on the part of the defendant to take care, and this duty must be one which is owed to the plaintiff himself, not merely to some indefinite group of people.†

The standard of care required of one who undertakes to perform an act is said to be the conduct of a "reasonable man." No one has been able to define "a reasonable man" which would satisfy all students of the law. Needless to say, the expression "reasonable man" is a fiction of the law, but a most valuable fiction. It provides a criterion by which human behavior may be evaluated. It will be noted that the behavior of men is expected to be guided by reason, or, as sometimes phrased, by prudence and care.[47]

> The general rule is that a "defendant charged with negligence can clear his feet" if he shows that he has acted in accord with the general and approved practice.[48]

It must be noted, however, that nurses and physicians may not always rely upon the defense that their conduct conformed to the general practice. A nurse charged with negligence cannot defend herself by by saying, "The nurses I work with always use this technique." Such a defense will be proper only when the general practice itself comports with the standard of care demanded of a reasonably prudent man. It has been cogently stated that

> ... neglect of duty does not cease by repetition to be neglect of duty.[49]

In the case of *McDaniel v. Vancouver General Hospital*,[50] the plaintiff, an infant, had been admitted to hospital with diphtheria. The child later contracted smallpox at the hospital. It was established that the technique of juxtaposing smallpox patients with others and of having a common nursing staff was the accepted practice. The trial resulted in a judgment for the plaintiff, which was reversed on ap-

---

*"The sound view, in my opinion, is that the law in all cases exacts a degree of care commensurate with the risk created."[43]

†Lord Justice Bowen pointed out: "The ideas of negligence and duty are strictly correlative and there is no such thing as negligence in the abstract; negligence is simply neglect of some care which we are bound to exercise toward somebody."[46]

peal. Though it has been said that a defendant charged with negligence can clear himself if he shows that he acted in accord with
general and approved practice, this must not be taken as inconsistent
with the general rule stated in the text. In this case, the plaintiff had
not proved that, in adopting the hospital technique described, the
defendant hospital was guilty of negligence. The decision rested
solely on the evidence.

An excellent summary of this subject was supplied by Justice
Adamson when he wrote:

> Negligence is shortly defined as the absence of care compared
> to the circumstances, and the general rule is that everyone is
> bound to exercise due care in his acts and conduct and omits or
> falls short of it at his peril. The standard is whether or not a
> person charged with negligence acted as a reasonable and prudent
> person would act. The test is whether a person charged with
> negligence has acted in such a way as reasonably could be
> required in such a case.[51]

When a nurse administered an overdose of a drug due to her
error in reading the physician's order, and as a consequence the
patient was injured, the nurse was held liable.[52]

Malpractice

Malpractice constitutes any professional misconduct, unreasonable lack of skill or fidelity in professional duties, evil practice, or
illegal or immoral conduct which results in injury or death to the
patient. To hold a physician or nurse responsible in damages, it must
be shown that the defendant failed to exercise the degree of skill and
care required by law. To be held liable, the evidence must reveal that
the professional conduct was not in accordance with the usual techniques of competent practitioners in the same field. In the United
States, the cases use the criterion of the standard of skill possessed by
the practitioners in the same locality. It would seem that in Canada a
reasonable degree of skill is expected of any practitioner.

> It has been held in some American cases that the locality in
> which the medical man practices is to be taken into account, and
> that a man practicing in a small village or rural district is not to
> be expected to exercise the high degree of skill of one having the
> opportunities afforded by a large city; and that he is bound to
> exercise the average degree of skill possessed by the profession in
> such localities generally. I should hestitate to lay down the law in
> that way; all the men practicing in a given locality might be
> equally ignorant and behind the times, and regard must be had to
> the present advanced state of the profession and to the easy means
> of communication with, and access to, the large centres of educa-
> tion and science.[53]

It bears repeating that malpractice suits stem from patients who
have poor results from treatment. Suits based on negligence or mal-

practice are entertained in the civil courts of Canada, and recovery has been allowed for numerous types of injuries.

Doctrine of *res ipsa loquitur*. Perhaps it is instructive at this point to explain the doctrine of *res ipsa loquitur*. As was mentioned above, the burden of proving negligence lies upon the plaintiff. The plaintiff is not required, however, to lay his finger on the exact negligent act on the part of the defendant, nor to isolate the specific act or omission which began the events leading to the injury. It is understandable that the plaintiff is wholly unable to allege just what act or omission caused his injury. He knows only that he was in the care of a particular nurse or physician. Consequently, the doctrine of *res ipsa loquitur* would be invoked by the plaintiff when he is unable to allege with any precision just what was the proximate cause of his injury or death (in the latter case, the suit is brought by next of kin or executrix). In other words, the Latin maxim is relied upon by an injured plaintiff whenever it is improbable that an accident would have happened had the defendant exercised due care. When there is reasonable evidence of negligence, and:

> . . . where the thing [causing the injury or death] is shown to be under the management of the defendant or his servants, and the accident is such as in the ordinary course of things does not happen if those who have the management use proper care, it affords reasonable evidence . . . that the accident arose from want of care.[54]

Obviously, when all the facts are in the possession of the plaintiff, there is no occasion for the application of this maxim. In such cases, the only question of law is whether the negligence can be inferred from the facts established.[55] There was a time when the doctrine of *res ipsa loquitur* was held not to apply in malpractice cases in Ontario.[56] More recently, however, it has been the tendency to apply the rule, depending upon the circumstances.[57]

The doctrine of *res ipsa loquitur* was held inapplicable in the case of *Morris v. Winsbury-White*.[58] In that case, the defendant agreed to perform a surgical operation upon the plaintiff. After the operation, the plaintiff remained in the hospital, attended by nurses and resident medical officers, although he was visited by the defendant-surgeon about three times a week. Tubes were inserted to drain the bladder, replacements being made by resident doctors and nurses. After his discharge it was found that a portion of a tube had been left in the plaintiff's bladder. In an action for both breach of contract and negligence, the court denied recovery, holding the doctrine inapplicable in the circumstances of the case.

Common Negligence Actions in Canada

The actions based on negligence in Canadian courts parallel the subject matter of negligence suits in American courts.

Failure to remove sponges. One of the most common acts of negligence in surgical cases has been the failure to remove sponges from an incision.[59] In *Jewison v. Hassard,* the defendant-surgeon removed a tube of pus from the abdomen of a patient by a surgical operation at a hospital. The tube broke, and the pus began to flow so fast that there was danger of its reaching the bowels and causing peritonitis. The defendant and another surgeon were compelled to swab out the cavity rapidly with gauze sponges, and removed, they thought, all the sponges as fast as they used them. When the swabbing was finished, the defendant inquired of the nurse whose duty it was to keep count of the sponges whether all the sponges were accounted for, and she replied in the affirmative. As it turned out, the wound did not heal well, owing to a gauze sponge which had been left in the wound. The court of appeal affirmed the trial court's judgment, which held that there was no negligence on the surgeon's part. The surgeon should be able to rely upon the nurse's count.[60] A contrary result was reached in an American case.[61]

Burns from faulty treatment. A content analysis of the decisions rendered by Canadian courts reveals further that burns resulting from faulty treatment give rise to many actions for damages. The burns may result from a routine matter, such as feeding a patient soup which proves to be too hot for consumption,[62] scalding from an inhalator or from diathermic treatment. In the case of *Sinclair v. Victoria Hospital,*[63] damages of $2000 against the hospital were awarded to a 15-month-old child who was severely scalded by a nickel-plated inhalator; the inhalator, full of boiling water, was so close to the infant's cot that by standing up in the crib and leaning over the side he could reach it. The nurse had left the child unattended. In another case, a hospital was held liable for serious burns to a patient as the result of the negligence of one of its nurses in putting an electric plug into the wrong socket upon administering a diathermic treatment, which was a part of her routine duty and not under the direction, control or supervision of a surgeon or physician, such treatment having been assumed by the hospital as part of its contract to nurse the patient. The appeal from an award of damages was dismissed.[64]

Mistakes in administering medications. Mistakes in administering medications are also serious grounds for litigation. A recent case involved a patient who dislocated his thumb and entered Harbour View Hospital for treatment. The attending physician directed an experienced graduate nurse to secure novocaine for a local anesthetic. The nurse asked another nurse for the drug, and the latter gave her a labeled bottle, but she failed to examine the label. The physician administered the solution; the patient died less than 30 minutes later. It appeared that the bottle contained a solution of Adrenalin. In entering a judgment for $10,000 against each of the nurses, the judge said:

In the case of drugs where the consequences of a mistake may be so grave, I think that anyone who is procuring a drug should use whatever means are within his power to prevent a mistake. It is true that as these matters become routine, there must be a tendency to expect that everything will be right but the nurse whose duty it was to provide the material for the work which the doctor was about to do, must, I think, have a duty to use the reasonable means at her disposal to make sure that she had the right drug. It was only a matter of looking at the label in this case and I must hold that she was negligent in not doing so.[65]

It should be noted that, although a hospital is liable for injury to a patient caused through the negligence of an employee during the regular course of her duties, the institution is not liable if the negligent act or omission does not belong to the kind of work for which that employee was engaged.[66]

Decisions Involving Acts of the Mentally Incompetent

Of interest to nurses and technicians serving in mental institutions in Canada are those decisions involving the acts of mentally incompetent persons. The case of *Crevier v. Hospital St. Luc*[67] involved a patient in a private hospital confined in isolation. The patient was under the supervision of nurses and male attendants, who bound him to the bed to prevent his escape. The patient managed to unbind himself, overpower the male attendant and jump through a window in a fit of madness. The court held that no negligence was attributable to the hospital, which was not answerable in damages for the patient's injuries.

A later case illustrates the trend to deny responsibility when the lunatic is incapable of appreciating the nature and consequences of his act and therefore is not liable in damages for his fault in causing injury to a nurse or attendant. The case in reference involved a suit brought by the widow of an attendant against the executors of a deceased lunatic. The patient, Zeron, was an elderly man who had suffered a severe cerebral hemorrhage followed by definite indicatons of senile dementia. The attending physician had warned the attendant that the patient was potentially a danger to others. The attendant was killed when the patient struck him with a piece of iron which the attendant had neglected to remove from the room. The trial court held that the negligence of the attendant was responsible for his death, and no liability attached to the lunatic therefor.[68] This holding, sustained on appeal, illustrates the principle of Canadian-American jurisprudence in this field of law that recognizes the defendant's *fault* rather than the plaintiff's damage as the predicate of liability.

The obligations of a hospital to a patient who manifests mental aberrations after entering the institution were set forth in an Ontario opinion which stands as the most recent pronouncement on the subject.[69] This case was an action by a husband and wife for damages due to injuries sustained by the latter while a patient in a hospital owned and operated by the defendants. The wife's actions in the hospital revealed that she was not normal mentally, and after a cesarean section had been performed, she was placed in a private room with a restraining jacket. A few days later she jumped out the window and sustained serious injuries. It was held that the nurses had no reason to anticipate a mishap which the doctors did not anticipate, and which appeared to have been unique in the experience of all the witnesses called at the trial. The plaintiff was a semiprivate patient, under the care of her own physician, and the responsibility of the hospital was simply to provide her with a room and bed, to bathe and feed her, to look to her comfort, to make routine observations as to temperature, pulse, and so forth, for the use of her doctor, and to carry out such special orders as the doctor might give. It was not part of the hospital's function, the court held, to make medical diagnoses or to lay down precautions for her safety (excepting in a case of obvious emergency).

Defects in Plant or Equipment

The importance to the nurse of bringing to the attention of the hospital authorities any defect in plant or equipment was the lesson taught by the case of *Bergeron v. Reilly and Chatham House Private Hospital.*[70] The plaintiff was a ward maid in a private hospital. She occupied a bedroom next to a fire escape. In cleaning her room, she went to the fire escape in order to shake out a scarf, and in so doing leaned over the rail of the fire escape and fell when it gave way. The plaintiff admitted that she knew before the accident that the rail was loose and had seen it hanging down at one end out of place. She did not report the defect to her employers, who testified that they were unaware of the condition despite periodic inspections. The action was dismissed, the court holding that the ward maid did not succeed in establishing a breach of duty on the part of the hospital. Moreover, the ward maid was contributorily negligent.

It has been held that a hospital is under a duty to provide fit and proper appliances for the treatment of its patients, and the standard here is the "usual and efficient appliances" in use at the time. It is not necessary that they should be the best available.[71]

Loss of or Damage to Patient's Property

The nurse's liability for the negligent loss of or damage to a patient's property is based upon her duty as a person to act as a reasonable and ordinary prudent person in handling such matters. The hospital is liable for any loss of the patient's property only when there is evidence to support a finding by a jury that the property was taken charge of by a nurse or other employee of the hospital.[72]

The Nurse as Anesthetist

In a Quebec case, the question was raised whether it is negligence *per se* for a trained nurse to serve as an anesthetist. It was settled in *Ducharme v. Royal Victoria Hospital*[73] that it was not negligence *per se* to have a trained nurse instead of a doctor as an anesthetist. The suit against the hospital was dismissed, as was the appeal.

Damages

What elements are taken into account in assessing damages against a defendant found to be negligent? The rationale of the law of damages is that damages should represent a monetary award, representing as nearly as possible compensation and indemnity for the loss sustained by the paintiff from the negligent act of the defendant. Damages are divided into two kinds, special and general. *Special* damages include hospital and doctor bills, loss of wages or salary, and other expenses which were unavoidably incurred by the injured party. *General* damages are usually difficult to calculate because they arise from such subjective claims as pain and suffering, loss of earning capacity, and more or less indiscrete claims based on curtailed physical activity. Permanent disability may be either partial or total, and damages are calculated upon the facts of the particular case. The factors which the court will weigh in assessing damages for permanent disability include the plaintiff's age and life expectancy, based upon actuarial tables, percentage of disability, and the plaintiff's earning capacity, based upon his employment record. Mr. Justice Bond noted that:

> . . . capacity to work of the injured party, his station in life; the nature of the work for which he is fitted; periods of enforced idleness; and ordinary risks of life and health should be considered.[74]

In view of the widespread popularity of private health insurance, it is interesting to note that insurance benefits are not to be considered when the jury or court assesses the damages in suits based upon injuries.*

At least one well-known Canadian nurse believes that each registered nurse should have her own liability insurance policy.[76] She also believes that the nursing practice act for each province should be

---

*As a matter of fact, Article 2468 of the Quebec Civil Code states that "civil responsibility shall in no way be lessened or altered by the effect of insurance contracts. . . ."[75]

reviewed to see whether it encompasses the work nurses are currently doing or whether they are practicing medicine in some situations. She also believes that Canadian nurses, like those in the United States, should seek the support of various professional organizations and joint statements of policy by them regarding the life-saving measures that may and do confront them in special care units.

TORTS AS A CAUSE OF OTHER CIVIL ACTIONS

Salmond, the distinguished authority on common law tort law, has defined a tort as:

> ... a civil wrong for which the remedy is a common law action for unliquidated damages, and which is not exclusively the breach of a contract or the breach of a trust or other merely equitable obligation.[77]

The remedies available for redress of a tort in an action at law are of three kinds, viz., damages, injunction, and specific restitution of property. Damages is the ordinary remedy, and the remedy most frequently sought in suits based on negligence which nurses are called upon to defend.

In Quebec, the term "delict" or "quasi-delict" is used instead of tort. The quasi-delict is due to an unintentional fault or negligence, whereas a delict is done with the intention of causing damage. A nurse in Quebec should read Article 1053 of the Civil Code.

A review of the case law reveals that Canadian jurisprudence recognizes the same groupings of legal wrongs for which a civil remedy exists as were outlined in the review of American law. Attention will be directed in the paragraphs which follow to those types of torts most frequently encountered by nurses.

Assault and Battery

A tort against which the nurse may be required to defend is assault and battery. The exact meaning and application of the term "assault and battery" are not well understood outside of legal circles. The definition of the expression will readily help the reader to understand why this is so. The tort consists of two aspects — an assault and a battery.

Battery. *Battery* is the application of force to the person of another without lawful justification. Technically, merely touching a person without his consent or some other lawful reason is actionable.[78] The rationale of the law on this subject is that not only is the individual to be free from bodily harm, but also that he shall be free from any form of insult due to interference with his person. Consequently, even when no physical harm results, a person may recover when his personal dignity or reputation is invaded by a battery.[79] Indeed, as Salmond points out:

> Intentionally to bring any material object into contact with another's person is a sufficient application of force to constitute a battery; for example, to throw water upon him, or to pull a chair from under him whereby he falls to the ground.[80]

There have been cases predicated upon battery when a person has been vaccinated against his will or when blood samples have been taken from him without his permission.

Assault. Turning now to the other aspect of the legal wrong, assault may be defined as the act of putting another person in reasonable fear of an immediate battery by means of an act amounting to an attempt or threat to commit a battery.[81] It is significant to note that the intent to do violence must be manifested in threatening acts and that merely insulting or menacing language alone is not enough.[82] It should be marked further that assault is not only a tort, but also a criminal offense, and that civil and criminal remedies may be pursued at the same time.*

Lack of consent for treatment or operation. Inasmuch as consent is a defense to a tort action in which a person is charged with intentionally interfering with either another person or his property, it is apparent that lack of consent or privilege is an integral element in establishing the legal wrong. But before a patient confers his consent for an operation or course of treatment, the implications of the proposed treatment or operation must be explained to him or to the person responsible for him. The law books are replete with cases of patients who sued for damages either because they did not consent to treatment or because they were not advised of the risks involved in the treatment.

By statute, in the Public Hospitals Act, express written consent except in an emergency is required for an operation in a public hospital.[84] And if the patient is an adult of sound mind, such consent is binding unless it is obtained by misrepresentation, fraud or duress.

EMERGENCY CASES. Generally speaking, a nurse or physician is not justified in projecting the treatment beyond the scope of the patient's consent on the alleged grounds that the treatment was urgently necessary.[85] Unauthorized extension of treatment or surgery is justified, nevertheless, in cases of emergency. "Emergency" may be defined as a situation imperiling the life or health of the patient. It is a question of fact in each case to determine whether or not an emergency exists. In a recent case, these definitions were given application. During a cesarean operation, the defendant surgeon dis-

---

*However, the Offences Against the Person Act, 1861, provides that summary criminal proceedings, whether they result in conviction or acquittal (after an actual hearing on the merits), are a bar to any subsequent civil proceeding for the same cause.[83]

covered a number of fibroid tumors in the uterus. After consulting with his assistant surgeon, he tied the plaintiff's fallopian tubes in order to prevent a second pregnancy, which would expose her to an extra hazard. It was held that the question for decision was not whether the time was convenient for the further operation without the plaintiff's consent, but whether such an emergency existed as made it necessary to do so. Since there was no evidence that the tumors were presently dangerous to health or life, the plaintiff was entitled to a judgment for trespass to her person, and $3000 damages were awarded.[86]

MINORS AND INCOMPETENTS. The importance of ascertaining whether or not the patient is old enough to confer his consent was illustrated by a case in which a patient entered the hospital for an operation on his nose.[87] He consented, on his own behalf, to the removal of part of an enlarged thyroid gland. It was later revealed that the patient, a youth of 19, of low intellect and subject to epileptic fits, was not capable of conferring his consent for the thyroid removal. Moreover, his parents were not notified by the hospital prior to the operation, and they brought an action against the hospital for trespass and assault. Though the action was dismissed on other grounds, it underscores the fact that not only must consent be conferred, but also that it must be conferred by one who is capable of giving it. The general rule is that if the person who consents is known to be an infant in the eyes of the law, mentally incompetent, or intoxicated — conditions which make a person incapable of giving consent — then the consent is not a valid defense in a suit. Needless to say, when the patient is a minor, the consent should be exacted from a parent or guardian; likewise in the case of an incompetent.*

Care of mentally disturbed patients. In Canada, laws governing hospitalization in psychiatric facilities are the business of the provincial legislatures. Recently, the trend has been toward more informality in admission. Further compulsory hospitalization of an unwilling person tends to be for a specified and limited period which may be continued only after the hospital authorities completely review his case and care. Swadron deplores the tendency of some to consider a person as either competent or incompetent for all purposes, and points out that many patients are competent to manage their affairs even though they need hospitalization.[88]

Since in Canada the field of criminal law and procedure is within the legislative area of the federal government, the care of a patient undergoing psychiatric treatment may be complicated by dealing

---

*Because of the views expressed in *Children's Memorial Hospital v. Davidson*,[90] in Quebec the father's consent should be obtained if at all possible without delaying the operation. The practice of the Province of Quebec is also unique in that consent forms require the husband's approval before an operation is to be performed on his wife, except in cases of legal separation.[91]

with two levels of government. Only through continuous inter-government cooperation can the problem be satisfactorily solved.[89]

A special, yet not infrequent, problem arises in the care and treatment of mentally disturbed patients. It is readily understandable that restraint may be called for in controlling such patients. There is, however, the possibility that legal action may be taken against the nurse or attendant if restraint is used unnecessarily or unskillfully. It will be recalled that threatening gestures accompanied by menacing words are sufficient to constitute a legal wrong known as assault. It follows that, except in emergencies, no actual restraint of any kind should be applied except on the direct order of a physician. Needless to say, when restraint is authorized, it should be carried out confidently, impersonally, and with the degree of skill demanded in the particular circumstances.[92]

Attention has been directed toward the liability of the nurse for assault and battery against the person or reputation of the patient. Conversely, the nurse may have a cause of action on the same grounds against the patient. And in this connection, it is well to remember that even children* and persons of unsound mind† are liable for their torts.

SELF-DEFENSE. It is well to remember that a trespass (attack) to the person may be justified on the grounds that one is acting in self-defense. This fact is of utmost importance in cases involving the care of mentally disturbed patients, in either public or private institutions, or in private homes. Consequently, a nurse who is attacked with a deadly weapon may defend herself with a deadly weapon or any other instrument which may protect her life. As pointed out in a leading case on the subject.

> He on whom an assault is threatened or committed is not bound to adopt an attitude of passive defence. He may lawfully take measures of aggression on his own account, so long as he does not go beyond what is reasonable as a measure of self-defence. Nor need he make any request or give any warning, but may forthwith reply to force with force.[94]

And it has been said that force is not reasonable if it is either unnecessary, i.e., greater than requisite for the purpose, or disproportionate to the evil to be prevented.[95]

False imprisonment. False imprisonment, or the unjustifiable detention of a person, or preventing a person from exercising his right

---

*"Minors. A minor is in general liable for his torts in the same manner and to the same extent as an adult. . . . A person under the age of 21 is in general free from all liability for breach of contract. In the law of torts, however, there are no similar rules of exemption. Thus, a child of any age may be sued for trespass to land or conversion, and will be held in damages just as if he were an adult" (*Salmond on the Law of Torts,* § 19).

†Insanity. "In wrongs of voluntary interference with the person, property, reputation, or other rights of other persons, such as trespass, assault, conversion, or defamation, it is no defence that the defendant is under an insane delusion as to the existence of sufficient legal justification. If he knew the nature and quality of his act, it is no defence that he did not know that what he was doing was wrong, whatever the position may be in the criminal law" (*Salmond on the Law of Torts,* § 20).[93]

of leaving the place in which he is may also subject a nurse to suit. Actions of this nature may arise when a nurse prevents a mentally disturbed patient from moving freely out of a room or building.[96] As under American law, a nurse in Canada may detain a patient long enough to ascertain whether a bill has been paid, but the period of time must be reasonable.

Defamation

Defamation is another wrongful action recognized by Canadian law. The wrong consists in the publication of a false and defamatory statement concerning a person without lawful justification.[97] The wrong of defamation may be either a libel or a slander.[98] Resultant legal action seeks to protect the interest which a person has in his reputation and good name. A nurse may sue a patient for defamation, and vice versa. Perhaps it is apposite to repeat the admonition at this point that the nurse should not discuss the ailments of her patients with persons not entitled to such information. Nor should she betray the other confidences obtained by virtue of her position.

Libel and slander. The common law recognizes a distinction between libel and slander in that libel is in all cases actionable *per se,* but slander is not actionable without proof of special damage, except in certain exceptional cases. The special damage spoken of must consist of the loss of a definite economic, material advantage. This is to say that slander must not consist merely in the loss of reputation itself.[99] Those exceptional cases in which slander is actionable *per se* without proof of special damage involve an imputation that the plaintiff has committed a criminal offense, that he suffers from a contagious social disease, or that the plaintiff (if a woman) is unchaste, or an imputation that reflects upon one's business, office or station in life.[100]

A defamatory statement may be legally excused or justified by showing that the person who made it was not moved to make it by a spirit of injury, but was motivated by a nonmalicious, justifiable purpose, for example, proof of consent, truth, privilege or fair comment. Of interest to the nurse is the defense of privilege. An authority on this aspect of the law has noted that privilege is of two kinds, absolute and qualified.

> A statement is said to be absolutely privileged when it is of such nature that no action will lie for it, however false and defamatory it may be, and even though it is made maliciously — that is to say, from some improper motive. Qualified privilege, on the other hand, exists when the defendant is exempted from the rule of strict liability, not absolutely, but only conditionally on the absence of malice.*

---

*Salmond on the Law of Torts, § 130. Absolute privilege covers statements made in judicial proceedings, parliamentary proceedings, offices of state, newspaper reports of public judicial proceedings, and parliamentary papers, and their republication in full.

Qualified privilege. Of particular interest to the nurse is that branch of the law known as qualified privilege.[101] The chief instances of qualified privilege are the following: when the nurse has a legal or moral duty to pass on information of a defamatory nature to another and when statements are made in the protection of an interest. As to the former, there are circumstances which impel a nurse to convey information of a degrading nature to another, such as to a physician or to the director of a nursing service. Perhaps the only guide for the nurse is to ask herself whether an ordinary, reasonable person under the circumstances would feel obliged to pass on derogatory information. As to the latter instance, protection of an interest, there are occasions which motivate a nurse to speak in self-defense. The occasions may arise from a charge against her of incompetence which rightly belongs upon the shoulders of a subordinate or fellow employee. Or the director of a nursing service, in the interests of candor, may have to report unfavorable aspects of the personal life of a nurse registered with the service.

Privileged communications. Before leaving the subject of defamation, mention should be made that although the doctor and nurse should not disclose information obtained from the patient in the course of the professional relationship, under Canadian law the obligation is not absolute and may give way when it is justified by public policy or there is a statute requiring a report of the matter. For example, The Public Hospitals Act requires reporting of the result of any Wassermann or Kahn test made on a sample of blood taken for a transfusion.[102]

An interesting case in which damages were recovered for defamation growing out of the application of the Venereal Disease Prevention Act is *The King v. Z.*[103] A physician employed by the Department of Health and Social Welfare in Quebec was asked to examine a patient. The doctor requested a nurse to make arrangements with the patient for the examination. The office of the nurse and the police station happened to be in the same building. The nurse, being a bit embarrassed, requested the Chief of Police to have the patient visit her office. After some messages, unfounded rumors made the rounds of the police station and the community that the patient was suffering from a venereal disease. When the rumors came to the patient's wife, she reacted by refusing to live with him until medical proof was offered her that he was free from any such disease. The patient sued the Government and recovered damages. This case appears to be sound law in Quebec, but there is some doubt as to whether it would be accepted as authoritative in a common law province. The reader will note that the case involves a provision of the Quebec statute itself which is read with the relevant section of the Civil Code.

Law Concerning Postmortem Examinations

It is advisable that the nurse practicing in Canada know something about the law concerning postmortem examinations. The Manitoba statute respecting coroners is typical of the statutory law on the subject. That statute reads, in part, as follows:

§ 5 In every case of violent or unnatural death, the coroner shall make an investigation into all the circumstances connected therewith and determine whether these are such that an inquest should or should not be held; and he shall report fully the result of his investigation to the Attorney-General.

§ 8 In the case of a sudden death from apparently natural causes, the coroner shall act on the request of the Attorney-General or a police officer.

§ 9 Where a coroner after investigation has good reason to believe that the deceased came to his death under circumstances calling for an inquest, he shall summon a jury and hold an inquest.

§ 29 (1) The coroner may at any time (a) for the purpose of an investigation; or (b) prior to the termination of an inquest by his order direct a post-mortem examination to be made by a medical practitioner with or without an analysis of the contents of the stomach and intestines.

(2) Where the coroner has reason to believe the death was directly or indirectly caused by the improper or negligent treatment of a medical examiner or other person, the medical practitioner or other person shall not be allowed to perform or assist at the post-mortem exam.[104]

Right of burial. In the absence of a testamentary disposition (a will) providing otherwise, the right to the possession of a dead body for the purpose of preservation and burial belongs to the surviving spouse or next of kin, and for any infraction of said right, such as an unlawful mutilation of the remains, an action for damages will lie. *Hunter v. Hunter* concerned a contest between members of an aged man's family after his death as to where he should be buried.[105] A son was named executor in his will, and letters probate had been granted him. In a suit against his mother and others, it was held that the executor had a right to the body for the purpose of burial, and an interim injunction was issued restraining the defendants from preventing the son from carrying out the burial.

Autopsy. In an action for interference with a corpse, recovery may include damages for mental suffering which results proximately from the wrongful act, even though no specific pecuniary damage is alleged or proved.[106] A case in point is *Philipps v. Montreal General Hospital,* in which the plaintiff-widow sued the defendant hospital for damages arising out of holding an autopsy on her late husband without her consent.[107] It was held that the allegations disclosed a cause of actions. However, a hospital is not liable in damages because the coroner performs a postmortem examination, following the report to him of the circumstances of the death of the patient, made with reasonable and probable cause by the chief intern of a hospital, notwithstanding the refusal of the widow to allow such examination.[108]

Acts Done at the Command of the Crown

Before leaving the subject of torts, it should be said that if a wrongful act has been committed against the person or property of any person, the wrongdoer cannot set up a defense that that act was done at the command of the Crown. It is a principle of common law jurisprudence that the Crown can do no wrong, and the Sovereign cannot be sued in tort, but the person who did the act is liable in damages as any private person would be. This rule of law, reiterated in a leading case in the House of Lords, is important when injuries are sustained in institutions operated by the Government or by its servants outside of hospitals.*[109]

Statutes of Limitation

It should be noted in passing that there may be provincial statutes which prescribe the period in which an action arising out of bodily injury or wrongful death may be brought. For example, the Quebec Civil Code, Article 2265(2), sets forth the prescription of one year in bodily injury actions, i.e., actions based in tort (delict or quasi-delict). However, when the action is based on contract rather than tort, the short prescription period of one year under the article is not applicable. The Public Hospital Act states:

> Any action against a hospital or any nurse or person employed therein for damages for injury caused by negligence in the admission, care, treatment or discharge of any patient shall be brought within six months after such patient is discharged from or ceases to receive treatment at such hospital and not afterwards.[111]

A malpractice suit against a physician must be commenced within one year from the date when the professional services giving rise to the alleged injury terminated.[112]

---

*Chief Justice Ritchie enunciated the law as follows: "In the contemplation of law, the Sovereign can do no wrong and is not liable for the consequence of her own personal negligence, so she cannot be made answerable for the tortious (negligent) acts of her servants. The doctrine of *respondeat superior* has no application to the Crown, it being the rule of the Common Law that the Crown cannot be prejudiced by the wrongful acts of any of its officers, for, as has been said long ago, no laches can be imputed to the Sovereign."[110]

After this decision had been rendered, the Dominion Government, by an amendment to the Exchequer Court Act in 1887, permitted actions to be brought against the Crown in the right of the Dominion for Negligence of its servants. The statute did not relieve the employee of the Crown of his own individual responsibility for his negligent or unlawful acts.

CRIMINAL MALPRACTICE, CRIMINAL NEGLIGENCE, AND WILLFUL VIOLATION OF POSITIVE LAW

Criminal acts refer to those acts or offenses against the public welfare or society as a whole, prosecuted in the name of the Crown. Under the law of Canada, nurses, like other persons, may subject themselves to criminal prosecution by doing anything or omitting to do anything which the Criminal Code of Canada specifies is an offense.

Definition of Criminal Acts

A broad definition of crime, while it may be appropriate in another country, cannot be used without qualification to the Criminal Code of Canada. The British North America Act, 1867, section 91, gives the power to the Parliament of Canada to make laws for the peace, order and good government of Canada in relation to all matters not coming within the classes of subjects assigned by the Act exclusively to the legislatures of the provinces, and includes, among other special categories, the criminal law, including the procedure in criminal matters.

In section 92, the Act assigns to the provincial legislatures a variety of subjects, including (paragraph 13) property and civil rights in the province. Section 92, paragraph 15, further provides for:

> . . . the imposition of punishment by fine, penalty, or imprisonment for enforcing any law of the province made in relation to any matter coming within any of the classes of subject enumerated in this section.

In consequence of this last provision, there are violations of provincial statutes punishable by fine or imprisonment which are not strictly speaking crimes in Canada, i.e., "infractions of the Criminal Code of Canada," but which nevertheless in a broad sense of the term might be considered crimes in other countries. The revised Criminal Code (1953-54) came into force in April, 1955.

Quebec, whose law in civil matters differs substantially from that of the other provinces, is governed, like all the other provinces, by the Criminal Code of Canada, which is a Dominion Statute.

Liability to Both Civil Suit and Criminal Action for Negligence

Ignorance of the law by a person who commits an offense is not an excuse. Nor does a person have to perform a wicked or immoral act before the law will regard the act as criminal. In another connection, the liability of a nurse for her negligent acts was discussed. It was mentioned, and bears repetition, that there are some acts of negligence so gross or wanton as to be regarded as criminal.

Criminal responsibility for acts just mentioned is set forth in the Criminal Code, 1953-54, Chapter 5.* It has been judicially held that to constitute criminal negligence the conduct must reach the level of gross negligence or wanton misconduct. Perhaps the liability has not been better delineated than by Associate Justice Grant:

> Whether the negligence in any case is of such a character as to justify conviction upon a criminal charge must depend upon the particular facts of the case itself. In order to found a criminal charge, there must be present such a degree of want of care as to involve a moral element; such a wanton or reckless indifference to the lives and safety of others, as would lead one to say, "The State should punish that man."[113]

Section 187 of the Criminal Code states:

> Everyone who undertakes to administer surgical or medical treatment to another person or to do any other lawful act that may endanger the life of another person is, except in cases of necessity, under a legal duty to have and to use reasonable knowledge, skill and care in so doing.

Thus, in *Rex v. Giardine,* it was held that a surgeon was not criminally negligent in administering a wrong drug to a patient when he had relied upon a nurse to supply him with the one he had requested.[114] In this case, a house surgeon was prosecuted on the ground that he should have examined the label on an ampule of diarsenol before administering it to a patient. This drug differs from Mapharsen and novarsan in that it must be neutralized before being injected, or it will cause the patient's death. The accused relied upon a graduate nurse to hand him the proper drugs. The negligence of both nurse and surgeon in not reading the label on the ampule before injecting the poisonous drug resulted in the death of the patient. The accused was acquitted, probably upon the testimony of expert witnesses who pointed out that experienced physicians rely to a large extent on the training of nurses. Such reliance, although resulting in tragic consequences, was not such culpable negligence as reached the level of gross negligence or wanton misconduct and disregard for life and limb.[115]

It will be recalled that a person may be subjected to both a civil suit and a criminal action arising from the same act or conduct.† The dual liability was succinctly pointed out by the Lord Chief Justice Hewart in *Rex v. Bateman,* wherein he noted that in a civil action for negligence the extent of a man's liability depends on how much

---

*Sec. 191(1) provides: "Everyone is criminally negligent who (a) in doing anything or (b) in omitting to do anything that is his duty to do, shows wanton or reckless disregard for the lives or safety of other persons." "(2) For the purpose of this section 'duty' means a duty imposed by law."

†"No civil remedy for an act or omission is suspended or affected by reason that the act or omission is a criminal offence" (*Martin's Criminal Code,* § 10).

damage he causes; in a criminal trial it depends on how negligent he was.[116] The question in the civil court is whether he was negligent;* the question in the criminal court is whether or not his negligence was so great as to be criminal—whether or not he went beyond a mere matter of compensation between subjects and showed such disregard for the life and safety of others as amounted to crime and deserved punishment.

Assault and battery. By way of illustration, reference may be made to the topic of assault and battery. It will be recalled that one may sue for the tort of assault and battery whenever someone applies force to the person of another without his consent. Even an attempt or threat, by act or gesture, to apply force to the person of another is actionable if such conduct causes the other to believe upon reasonable grounds that present ability exists to effect the harmful purpose.[118] Such behavior is also criminal.[119] A physical examination of a woman who was being held upon a charge of concealment of birth was made by a physician pursuant to an order of a magistrate. The woman had not given her consent. The act of the physician was held to be an assault.[120]

Penalties. The penalties for the crime of criminal negligence are severe in Canada. One who by criminal negligence causes bodily harm to another person is guilty of an indictable offense and is liable to imprisonment for 10 years; if one's criminal negligence results in death, the penalty upon the finding of guilt is imprisonment for life.[121]

Possession and Dispensing of Narcotics

Unless a nurse has some knowledge of the constitutional position of Canada with respect to the subject of the food and drug law, the variety of statutes is apt to be confusing. The Government has exercised care in such legislation as the Food and Drug Act and the proprietary or Patent Medicines Act so as not to treat any phase of the handling of narcotic drugs.

The first measure in narcotic regulation was an act of Parliament in 1908 dealing with the suppression of opium.[122] Further legislation was enacted in 1911, bringing cocaine, morphine and heroin under control. In 1919, a Federal Department of Health was created, and to it was assigned the administration and supervision of the enforcement of the Narcotic Act of 1920, a landmark statute on the subject.[123] A Narcotic Division was formed within the Department of Health, today the Department of National Health and Welfare. By definition, a narcotic drug is any substance mentioned in the Schedule

---

*The degree of the negligent conduct is not the measure of the damages due. In *St. Onge v. Bernier,* the negligence was held to be extremely slight, yet the dental surgeon was made to pay damages.[117]

of the Act. The Schedule includes not only opium and its derivatives, but also the newer synthetic drugs. The Schedule requires amendment from time to time to include such newer synthetic drugs as they appear on the market.

Judicially, it has been stated that the Opium and Narcotic Drug Act contains the entire code for legal as well as the illegal use of narcotic drugs. The administration of the Opium and Narcotic Drug Act is by statute the responsibility of the Department of National Health and Welfare; but by arrangement with the Royal Canadian Mounted Police the enforcement of the statute is a responsibility of that group. Legal agents specially appointed by the Department of Justice handle the prosecution of offenses under the Act through the Department of National Health and Welfare.

A license from the Minister of National Health and Welfare, approved by the Governor in Council, is necessary for the commercial handling of narcotic drugs by wholesalers. An elaborate scheme of periodic audits of the books and records of hospitals and retail druggists as to their supplies and use of narcotic drugs is conducted by a diligent staff of the Department of National Health and Welfare, aided by specially trained officers of the Royal Canadian Mounted Police. Doctors, dentists and veterinary surgeons, while not required by the Act to keep as detailed records, may nevertheless be required to furnish explanations by the department concerning their purchase and distribution of narcotic drugs.

The nurse may be held liable for violating the Opium and Narcotic Drug Act. Heavy penalties are imposed for the illegal possession, distribution, transportation, and so on, of narcotic drugs.[124]

When the accused is proved to have been in physical possession or control of a drug, it is no defense for him to say that he did not know that the substance in his possession was a drug. Indeed, liability to conviction is placed upon the occupier of the premises in which the drug is found.* This aspect of absolute liability was clearly set forth in *R. v. Ryan*.[126] The accused was tried for unlawful possession of drugs. The jury returned a verdict of "guilty without criminal intent," which they clarified to mean that the accused:

> . . . had no intentions of converting it to his own use or selling it.

In construing this as a guilty verdict, Justice Graham observed:

> S. 4(1)(d) has been before the Courts of Canada many times, and it is established that nothing more than proof of possession is necessary to constitute an offence under it. . . .

In Quebec, only physicians licensed and in good standing within the Medical Act of 1925 may dispense narcotics as drugs.† No special

---

*Ignorance of the nature of the substance was held not to avail as a defense.[125]

†A physician who failed to pay his annual contributions to the College of Physicians, and was not therefore in good standing under the law, could not invoke the provisions of the Opium and Narcotic Drug Act of 1929 when prosecuted thereunder.[127]

registration for this purpose is required, as in the United States. A nurse may not legally be in possession of narcotics unless she is administering them to a patient on a doctor's order, or she is herself a patient for whom the physician has prescribed them, or is the official custodian of the narcotics in a hospital department.[128]

Abortion or Procurement of Miscarriage

It is necessary to discuss the subject of abortion or procurement of miscarriage under this section dealing with criminal malpractice. Under the Canadian Criminal Code, a person is guilty of abortion if he:

> ... with intent to procure the miscarriage of a female person, whether or not she is pregnant, uses any means for the purpose of carrying out his intention. . . .[129]

A penalty may be imposed as severe as imprisonment for life. The term "means," as used in this section of the Code, includes (a) the administration of a drug or other noxious thing, (b) the use of an instrument, and (c) manipulation of any kind. It is also a crime to supply anyone or to procure unlawfully a drug or other noxious thing to be used to procure a miscarriage.[130]

As was just pointed out, the act committed is an offense whether or not the woman is pregnant at the time the attempt is made to induce an abortion.[131] Even if the woman does not take any of the substance supplied her to induce an abortion, if such was the intent of the supplier, an offense was committed. Such was the holding in *R. v. Pettibone,* wherein Justice Stuart, delivering the judgment, said:

> Now even if the doctor deceived the accused and gave him innocuous material yet if the accused really tried, as I think the jury could reasonably infer that he did, to get a noxious material, believed that he had got it and tried to get the woman to take it, in my view there was much more than mere preparation, there was a real attempt to commit the offence and the fact that owing to the doctor's deceit it was impossible for him to commit it, would not make any difference.[132]

In this case, the conviction was for an *attempt* to commit a violation of Section 303, now Section 237(1). The woman, the intended victim, had not yet taken any of the substance, and there was no analysis to prove what it was.

When an *attempt* to perform an illegal abortion results in the death of the woman, the physician, nurse or other party who performed the operation is subject to conviction for murder, if he or she knew or should have known that death was likely to ensue. If the physician, nurse or other party did not know or could not have known that the act was likely to cause death, a conviction of manslaughter may follow. The latter was the verdict in the publicized case of *R. v. Azoulay.*[133] The accused was charged with the murder of Blanche Lepire. The Crown contended that the defendant-appellant, for the unlawful purpose of procuring a miscarriage of the deceased woman, used on her instruments which eventually caused her death. The defense was that at the moment the accused was about to examine the woman internally for fibromas, a spontaneous process of miscarriage started, causing severance of the placenta from the wall of the uterus and leading to a fatal hemorrhage. Was the rupture natural, or had it been provoked artifically by the accused physician with the intent of bringing about an abortion? The verdict of manslaughter was upheld by the court of appeal, but later set aside by the Supreme Court of Canada on the ground of inadequacy in the judge's charge to the jury. At the new trial, the Crown Prosecutor's remarks resulted in declaring a mistrial. At the third trial, in November, 1955, the physician was found guilty of manslaughter and drew a sentence of six years.

Needless to say, consent of the patient to undergo a criminal abortion is no defense.

THE NURSE AS WITNESS IN COURTS OF JUSTICE

The professional activities of the average nurse sometimes make it necessary that she testify in open court on some matter of which she has direct or circumstantial evidence. The nurse may be summoned to appear in court either by the parties to a civil action or by the Crown or the defendant in a criminal prosecution. By way of illustration, the nurse may be called upon to testify as to the mental condition of a testator at the time of making a will;* the insanity of a prisoner-patient accused of a crime;[136] the time and cause of a death; whether or not an abortion was performed ar attempted; in bodily injury cases, and many other matters.

Duties and Qualifications of a Witness

It should be understood that a witness is under a duty to do all that he or she can do to assist the course of justice. A recent article in the leading law journal of Canada sets forth the qualities of the effective witness with the following words:

> No complete description of the good witness can be given, but, generally speaking, the forthright individual who speaks clearly and answers only the questions asked of him makes by far the best impression. Be attentive to questions, particularly in cross-examination. Answer them briefly and where possible without using medical terms. I have seen juries sit up expectantly when a doctor is called to the witness box and then gradually lose interest as he

---

*The law requires a "sound, disposing mind" on the part of the testator in order for a will to be valid. An interesting recent case which delineates the necessary prerequisites is *Re Sample*.[134] The previous landmark case was *Robins v. National Trust Co., Ltd.*[135]

proceeds to describe the case in technical language. He might as well have been speaking in a foreign language. Not only is the attention of the jury lost; but jurymen, and sometimes even judges, are irritated by being asked to listen to what they cannot understand.

It is never wise to volunteer information. A volunteered answer usually leads to trouble, and sometimes to disaster.

Do not lose your temper. I have often seen a witness make a good impression through a long examination only to destroy it in the last few minutes by losing his temper at what he considers to be some inane question or a personal affront. Usually, he retires from the witness box having injured the case.[137]

Before the witness offers his testimony, an oath is administered in which he affirms to tell the truth, the whole truth and nothing but the truth. Perjury is punishable under criminal jurisprudence. As to the witness subjecting himself to an action for damages when he makes a defamatory statement in evidence, the Ontario and Canada Evidence Acts state that:

> A witness shall not be excused from answering any question upon the ground that the answer may tend to ... establish his liability in a civil proceeding at the instance of the Crown or of any person.[138]

An authority on the subject points out that:

> ... the privilege of a witness to refuse to answer a question when the answer tends to incriminate himself, which had been recognized by the common law and statutes for a long time was abolished in criminal cases by the Canada Evidence Act of 1893, and in civil cases by the Ontario Evidence Act of 1904.[139]

In brief, under the Canada Evidence Act a witness may not refuse to answer a question when the answer tends to incriminate him. His recourse is to ask the court to protect him under the Canada Evidence Act; then he must answer the question, but his answer may be used against him only on a charge of perjury in the giving of that evidence. It is instructive to note at this point that the Canada Evidence Act applies only to criminal and civil proceedings in which the Parliament of Canada has jurisdiction. A witness giving evidence in proceedings held pursuant to a provincial statute receives no protection other than that afforded by provincial law.[140]

Under Canadian law, a nurse is not authorized to give medical opinions either before a case is brought to court or in testimony at trial. However, like any witness in the witness box, a nurse may state what she has seen, heard or done.[141] The nurse is not qualified to testify as an expert on the practice of medicine.[142]

REFERENCES

1. Fidler and Gray: *Law and the Practice of Nursing,* 1947. Professor Corry: *Elements of Democratic Government,* 1947 (contrasts British, Canadian and

American governmental systems). The British North America Act, 1867, 30 Vict. c. 3: Distribution of Legislative Powers VI, § 91-95

2. Walton: *Scope and Interpretation of the Civil Code of Lower Canada.* 1907, pp. 5, 23

3. Payne, Julien D.: Law and the Canadian Position. *Nurs. Clin. N. Am.,* 2 (1) 161-173, Mar., 1967

4. Wright: What Is a Profession? 29 *Can. Bar Rev.,* 748 (1951). See also Macmillan (Lord): *Law and Other Things.* 1938, p. 127

5. Kitchen: *Law for the Medical Practitioner.* p. 145

6. [1904] 2 K.B. 602 (Eng.), 73 L.J.K.B. 819, 13 Mews 666

7. Frere v. Shields [1939] 3 D.L.R. 265, 2 W.W.R. 396 (Sask. C.A.) (immoral consideration); Hardman v. Falk, 15 W.W.R. (N.S.) 337, [1955] 3 D.L.R. 129, affirming [1955] 1 D.L.R. 432 (B.C.C.A.) (mental incompetent); Casavant v. Ashby, 44 Rev. Leg. 373 (n.s.) (Que., 1938) (lack of consent); Spalding v. Donald, [1943] O.W.N. 379, aff'd, [1943] O.W.N. 702 (undue influence)

8. R.S.A. 1942, c. 184 s. 13 (1) b

9. [1946] 2 W.W.R. 536, [1946] 3 D.L.R. 707 (Alta.)

10. Cf. Edmonton Hospital Board v. Jones, [1950] 1 W.W.R. 651, [1950] 1 D.L.R. 772 (Atla. C.A.), in which the court held that the Hospitals Act was not to be construed to mean that the husband was not to be protected under a legal separation granted under the Domestic Relations Act, R.S.A. 1942, c. 300, s. 12

11. [1946] O.W.N. 884 (Ont. C.A.). See also Fortin v. Fortin, (1916) 49 C.S. 267 (Que.) (special services implies extra compensation)

12. Allen v. Froh [1932] 1. W.W.R. 593 (Sask.)

13. See Meunier v. L'Heureux, (1935) 74 C.S. 460 (Que.) (dentist in arrears under Quebec Dentists' Act, 1925). For litigation involving illegal practice of medicine, see Quebec College of Physicians and Surgeons v. Fortin (1936) 74 C.S. 111 (Que.); Lesage v. Quebec College of Physicians and Surgeons (1936) 60 B.R. 1 (Que.) 65 Can. C.C. 392, [1936] 3 D.L.R. 71 modifying 71 C.S. 338, (Que. C.A.); Quebec College of Physicians and Surgeons v. Tapp (1936) 74 C.S. 218 (Que.). To constitute the practice of medicine, there must be a course of conduct. An isolated act is insufficient to justify a conviction for illegal practice. Collège des Médecins et Chirurgiens de Québec v. Fortin [1944] C.S. 266 (Que.), applied in College of Physicians v. Saucier, 80 Can. C.C. 245, (1943) Can. Abr. 587

14. *Salmond on the Law of Torts,* § 149. (Pentecost v. London District Auditor [1951] 2 K.B. 759, 764, [1951] 2 All E.R. 330)

15. See Lord Wright in Caswell v. Powell Duffryn Associated Collieries, Ltd. [1940] A.D. 152, 175-6; [1940] A.C. 152; [1939] 3 All E.R. 722; 108 L.J.K.B. 779; 55 T.L.R. 1004; 161 L.T. 374

16. Seare v. Prentice (1807) 8 East. 348; 173 Eng. Rep. 581

17. (1838) 8 C. and P. 475 at 479, 173 Eng. Rep. 581. Quoted with approval in Town v. Archer (1902) 4 O.L.R. 383

18. The rule was recognized and applied in Robe & Clothing Co. v. Kitchener (1923) 55 O.L.R. 1 varied [1925] S.C.R. 106, [1925] 1 D.L.R. 1165. See also Dimitroff v. Gonder (1924) 56 O.L.R. 119.

19. Winn v. Alexander [1940] 3 D.L.R. 778, [1940] O.W.N. 238

20. Mellen v. Nelligan [1952] C.S. 446 (Que.)

21. C. v. C. [1946] 1 All E.R. 562

22. (1916) 10 W.W.R. 45, 22 B.C. 405, 27 D.L.R. 235 (B.C. C.A.)

23. Davis v. Colchester Co. Hospital Trust, (1933) 7 M.P.R. 66, [1933] 4 D.L.R. 68 (C.A. N.S.)

24. Fidler and Gray: *Law and the Practice of Nursing,* pp. 59-60. Smith, Alice: Nurses Working Alone in Rural Areas. *Canadian Nurse,* 50:965-7 (1954)

25. Fidler and Gray: *op. cit. supra.* note 24, p. 61

26. On the general subject of tort liability, see Thomson: *Law of Negligence and Delicts in Canada,* 1946, and *Salmond on the Law of Torts,* 10th ed, Sec. 3, 31, 32, 35, 41. Illustrative cases include Hewitt v. Bonvin [1940] 1 K.B. 188 (Eng.) (servant defined); Warren v. Henleys, Ltd., [1948] 2 All E.R. 935 (master-servant relation); Young v. Edward Box & Co., [1951] 1 T.L.R. 789 (Eng.) (vicarious liability); Performing Right Society, Ltd. v. Mitchell and Booker, Ltd., [1924] 1 K.B. 762 (Eng.) (independent contractor distinguished from servant)

27. Vancouver General Hospital v. Fraser [1951] 4 D.L.R. 736, affirmed by [1952] 2 S.C.R. 36

28. Cassidy v. Minister of Health [1951] 2 K.B. 343.

29. See also Swanson, A. L.: Some Legal Responsibilities in Hospitals. *Canadian Nurse,* 50:958-61 (1954)

30. Petite v. Macleod *et al.,* [1955] 1 D.L.R. 147 (N.S. Sup. Ct.)

31. Illustrative cases include Hall v. Lees, *supra,* note 6; Lavere v. Smith's Falls Public Hospital (1915) 35 O.L.R. 98, 26 D.L.R. 346 reversing 34 O.L.R. 216, 24 D.L.R. 866 (C.A.). In the latter case, Justice Riddell stated: "There can be no possible doubt that the burn was caused by an over-heated brick being placed against the foot of the anaesthetised and unconscious patient; that this was done by the nurse in charge; and that such an act was improper. There can be no doubt of the liability of the nurse civilly in tort, unless she can justify herself by a command of someone she was bound to obey; but the nurse is not sued here. The sole question is whether the hospital is liable for the act of the nurse."

32. [1935] 2 D.L.R. 804, [1935] 1 W.W.R. 651 (Alta.). Bernier v. Sisters of Service, [1948] 2 D.L.R. 468

33. (1907) 10 O.W.R. 876

34. R.S.O. 1897, c. 248

35. [1926] 1 W.W.R. 36, [1926] 1 D.L.R. 91 (Alta.)

36. Vuchar v. Trustees of Toronto General Hospital [1937] 1 D.L.R. 298, [1937] O.R. 71, [1936] O.W.N. 589, reversing [1936] 3 D.L.R. 221, [1936] O.R. 387, [1936] O.W.N. 350. In Nyberg v. Provost Municipal Hospital [1927] S.C.R. 266, [1927] 1 D.L.R. 969, reversing [1926] 1 W.W.R. 890, 22 Alta. 1, [1926] 2 D.L.R. 563, Anglin, C.J.C., wrote: "I regard the failure of the nurse . . . to make sure that the hot water bottle against his leg was not a source of danger, as inexcusable and as negligence in her capacity as a servant of the hospital corporation in a matter of ministerial ward duty, if not mere routine, which entailed responsibility on that body for its consequences. The obligation undertaken by the hospital authority (apart from the operation itself and the services of surgeons and nurses in the operating room) was not merely to supply properly qualified nurses, but to nurse the plaintiff [Hall v. Lees, *supra*]. It is negligence of their servant in the discharge of that contractual obligation that caused the severe injury of which the plaintiff complains." See also Guild, D. J.: The Promotion of Safety. *Canadian Nurse,* 51:456-9 (1955)

37. Barker v. Lockhart [1940] 3 D.L.R. 427, 14 M.P.R. 546 (N.B. C.A.). Accord, Craig Bros. v. Sisters of Charity [1940] 4 D.L.R. 561, [1940] 3 W.W.R. 336 (Sask. C.A.) affirming D.L.R. *loc. cit.* [1940] 2 W.W.R. 80

38. Petit v. Hospital Ste. Jeanne d'Arc, (1940) 78 C.S. 564 (Que.)

39. Petite v. Macleod *et al., supra,* note 30. See also Cassidy v. Ministry of Health, [1951] 2 K.B. 343, [1951] 1 All E.R. 574 (Eng.)

40. Roe v. Minister of Health [1954] 2 Q.B. 66, [1954] 2 All E.R. 131 (Eng.)

41. *Salmond on the Law of Torts,* (10th ed.) p. 85

42. Gebbie v. Saskatoon [1930] 2 W.W.R. 625, 25 Sask. 7, 41 Can. Ry. Cases 45, [1930] 4 D.L.R. 543 (C.A.) per Martin, J. A., quoting Alderson, B in Blyth v. Birmingham Waterworks Co., (1856) 11 Ex. 781 at 784, 156 Eng. Rep. 1047. Another early case, Grill v. General Iron Screw Collier Co., (1866) L.R. 1 C.P. 600, 612 (Eng.), defined negligence as "the absence of such care as was the duty of the defendant to use."

43. Lord Macmillan in Read v. J. Lyons & Co. [1947] A.C. 156, at 173. For a similar approach in the criminal law, see The People v. Dunleavy [1948] Ir. R. 95 (Ire.) (manslaughter)

44. Levi v. Colgate-Palmolive (1941) 41 S.R. (N.S.W.) 48, aff'd. 65 C.L.R. 663 (Austr.). See also *Salmond on the Law of Torts,* § 147

45. O'Brien v. Michigan Central Ry., (1909) 19 O.L.R. 345 (C.A.) See also *Salmond on the Law of Torts,* § 150

46. *In re* Thomas v. Quartermaine (1887) Q.B.C. 685, 694, 56 L.J.Q.B. 340, 3 T.L.R. 495, 57 L.T. 537 (C.A.). Cf. McAlister or Donoghue v. Stevenson [1932] A.C. 562, 618, 147 L.T. 281, 48 T.L.R. 494 per Lord Macmillan

47. See discussion by Chief Justice Tindal in Vaughan v. Menlove (1837) 3 Bing. N.C.

486, 495, 132 Eng. Rep. 490 (Ct. of C.P.) and by Alderson, B., in Blyth v. Birmingham Waterworks Co., *op cit.,* note 41

48. Vancouver General Hospital v. McDanial (1934) 152 L.T. 56 at 57, per Lord Alness

49. Lord Tomlin in Bank of Montreal v. Dominion Guarantee Co., [1930] A.C. 659 at 666

50. McDaniel v. Vancouver General Hospital [1934] 3 W.W.R. 619, [1934] 4 D.L.R. 593 reversing [1933] 3 W.R.R. 447, 41 Man. 570

51. Ratcliffe v. Whitehead, [1933] 3 W.W.R. 447, 41 Man. 570

52. Strangeways v. Lesmere v. Clayton [1936] 2 K.B. 11

53. Town v. Archer *et al.,* (1902) 4 O.L.R. 383 (Ont.)

54. Scott v. London and St. Katherine's Docks Co., (1865) 3 H & C. 596 at 601, 159 Eng. Rep. 665

55. Barkway v. South Wales Transport Co., [1950] 1 All E.R. 392, 395 (Eng.) See the thorough treatment of this topic by Underhay, 14 *Can. Bar Rev.,* 287-94 (1936); also Lewis: A Ramble with *Res Ipsa Loquitur* (1951) 11 *Camb. L. J.* 74

56. Hughston v. Jost [1943] 1 D.L.R. 402 (Ont.)

57. Nesbitt v. Holt [1953] 1 S.C.R. 143, 1953 1 D.L.R. 671, affirming judgment of the Ontario Court of Appeal [1951] O.W. 601, [1951] 4 D.L.R. 478

58. Morris v. Winsbury-White [1937] 4 All E.R. 494 (Eng.)

59. X v. Raiotte (1938) 64 B.R. 484 (Que.) affirming 74 C.S. 569 (Que.) 1937 Can. Abr. 635; Meyer v. Lefebvre [1942] 1 D.L.R. 668, [1942] 1 W.W.R. 485 (Alta. C.A.) (although damage resulted from a quantity of gauze left in the incision, the jury held that the negligence consisted in failure to use x-ray equipment, and the case was remanded for a new trial)

60. Jewison v. Hassard (1916) 28 D.L.R. 584 (Man. C.A.)

61. Stawicki v. Kelly, 113 N.J. 556, 174 Atl. 896 (1934)

62. Wyndham v. Trustees of Toronto Gen'l Hospital [1938] 1 D.L.R. 797, [1938] O.W.N. 55, in which the plaintiff recovered a judgment of $4000 plus costs

63. Sinclair v. Victoria Hospital [1943] 1 D.L.R. 302, [1943] 1 W.W.R. 30, 50 Man. 297, aff'g. [1942] 4 D.L.R. 652, [1942] 3 W.W.R. 273, Man. *loc. cit.*

64. Sisters of St. Joseph v. Fleming [1938] 2 D.L.R. 417, [1938] S.C.R. 172, aff'g. [1937] 2 D.L.R. 121, [1937] O.R. 512 [1937] O.W.N. 207

65. Bugden v. Harbour View Hosp. [1947] 2 D.L.R. 338 (N.S.C.A.) See also Challener: Rights, Liabilities and Duties of a Professional Nurse. 54 *Dickinson L. Rev.* 280-92 (1950)

66. The principle is discussed in Sheehan v. Bank of Ottawa, (1923) 35 B.R. 432 (Que.)

67. Crevier v. Hospital St. Luc, 46 *Rev. de Jur.* 459 (Que., 1940)

68. Wilson v. Zeron [1942] 2 D.L.R. 580, [1942] O.W.N. 195

69. Flynn v. Hamilton and Governors of Hamilton City Hospital [1950] O.W.N. 224, reversing [1948] O.W.N. 855, 1948 Can. Abr. 317 (Ont. C.A.)

70. Bergeron v. Reilly and Chatham House Private Hospital (1945) 62 B.C. 208

71. Moore *et al.* v. Large [1932] 2 W.W.R. 568 (B.C.C.A.)

72. Gumina v. Toronto Gen. Hosp. Trustees (1920) 19 O.W.N. 547 (C.A.). Although the plaintiff had a verdict returned in his favor by the trial jury, it was reversed on appeal for the reason cited in the text.

73. Ducharme v. Royal Victoria Hospital (1940) 69 B.R. 162 (Que.), affirming 76 C.S. 309 (Que., 1940)

74. Robbin v. Frechette (1931), 51 B.R. 514, 515 (Que.)

75. 6 Geo. VI, c. 68. For cases involving automobile collision and liability insurance, see Hebert v. Rose (1935) 58 B.R. 459 (Que.); also Jackson v. Joel and Wilkins [1947] 2 W.W.R. 659, [1948] 1 W.W.R. 156 (Sask. C.A.).

76. Crotin, Gloria G.: Medicolegal Problems Can Arise in the Coronary Care Unit. *Canad. Nurse,* 65: 37-9, April, 1969

77. *Salmond on the Law of Torts,* § 3. See also Wright: The Law of Torts: 1923-1947. 26 *Can. Bar Rev.,* 46 (1948); Williams: The Aims of the Law of Torts. [1951] *Current Legal Problems,* 157; Williams: The Foundations of Tortious Liability. 7 *Camb. L.J.* 111 (1939)

78. Cole v. Turner, (1704) 6 Mod. 149, 87 Eng. Rep. 907 (Nisi Prius) per Holt, C. J.

79. Dumbell v. Roberts [1941] 1 All E.R. 326 (a man's fingerprints taken without his consent before he has been committed for trial)

80. *Salmond on the Law of Torts,* § 111, citing Pursell v. Horn, (1838) 8 Ad. & E. 602, 112 Eng. Rep. 966, and Hooper v. Reeve, (1817) 7 Taunt. 698, 129 Eng. Rep. 278
81. Covell v. Laming (1808) 1 Camp. 497, 170 Eng. Rep. 1034; Eisener v. Maxwell [1951] 1 D.L.R. 816
82. Meade's and Belt's Case, (1823) 1 Lew. 184, 168 Eng. Rep. 1006
83. See Turner: Assault at Common Law. *Modern Approach to Criminal Law,* p. 344
84. R.R.O. 1960, Reg. 523, Sec. 42
85. Parmley v. Parmley and Yule [1945] S.C.R. 635 at 645; [1945] 4 D.L.R. 81
86. Murray v. McMurchy [1949] 2 D.L.R. 442, [1949] 1 W.W.R. 989 (B.C. Sup. Ct.)
87. Booth v. Toronto General Hospital (1910) 17 O.W.R. 118
88. Swadron, Barry B.: Legal Problems in Care of Mentally Ill. *Canadian Nurse,* 61:895, Nov., 1965
89. *Idem.*
90. Children's Memorial Hospital v. Davidson (1936) 74 C.S. 268 (Que.)
91. *Cf.* Lalumière v. X, [1946] C.S. 294 (Que.); Art. 986a C.C.
92. See Fidler and Gray: *Law and the Practice of Nursing,* Chap. 5, "Mental Illness."
93. Morriss v. Marsden, [1952] 1 All E.R. 925 (person of unsound mind liable for assault and battery)
94. Green v. Goddard, (1704) 2 Salk. 641, 91 Eng. Rep. 540. See also Turner v. M-G-M Pictures, Ltd., [1950] 1 All E.R. 449
95. Leward v. Baseley (1695) 1 Ld. Raym. 62, 91 Eng. Rep. 937
96. The article by Amos: Contractual Restraint of Liberty, 44 *L.Q.R.,* 464 (1928), is instructive on this topic. For the action arising from false arrest, see Warner v. Riddiford (1858) 4 C.B. (N.S.) 180, 140 Eng. Rep. 1052 (Common Pleas)
97. See Wade: Defamation. 66 *L.Q.R.* 348 (1950); also Lloyd: Reform of the Law of Libel. [1952] *Current Legal Problems,* 168
98. Weber v. Birkett [1925] 1 K.B. 720; [1925] 2 K.B. 152
99. Roberts v. Roberts (1864) 5 B. & S. 384, 122 Eng. Rep. 874
100. Gray v. Jones (1939) 160 L.T. 361 (Eng.) (criminal offense imputed); Bloodworth v. Gray (1864) 7 Man. & C. 334, 135 Eng. Rep. 140 (venereal disease imputed); Kerr v. Kennedy [1942] 1 K.B. 409 (Eng.) (unchastity against a woman); Brown v. Smith (1853) 13 C.B. 596, 138 Eng. Rep. 1333 (reflecting upon plaintiff's business or office). A unique case, interesting because of its implications, is Brunelle v. Girard, (1914) 23 B.R. 427 (Que.), in which it was held that the publication in a newspaper of an article tending to defame an author and suggesting that he was a Freemason, in a center of Roman Catholic population, was a libel
101. See Defamation Act, 1952, Sec. 7, dealing with privileged statements; also Goodhart: Defamatory Statements and Privileged Occasions. 56 *L.Q.R.,* 262 (1940)
102. R.S.O. 1960, Ch. 322. Reg. 522, Sec. 48. See Fleming, Meredith, and Joyce, Terrence, C. R.: Privileged Communication Between Physician and Patient. *Canad. Hosp.,* 45:41-3, July, 1968
103. The King v. Z [1947] B.R. 457 (Que.)
104. R.S.M. 1954, c. 46, "An Act Respecting Coroners." For similar statutes in other provinces, consult R.S.Q. 141, c. 22, s. 25, c. 265, s. 4; R.S.N.B. 1952, c. 41; R.S.S., 1953, c. 106
105. Hunter v. Hunter (1930) 65 O.L.R. 586
106. Edmonds v. Armstrong Funeral Home, Ltd., 25 Alta. 173 [1930] 3 W.W.R. 649 (postmortem performed without consent)
107. Philipps v. Montreal General Hospital (1908) 33 C.S. 483 (Que.) (containing a review of the common law and civil law with Canadian practice).
108. Religieuses Hospitalières de l'Hotel-Dieu de Montréal v. Brouilette [1943] B.R. 441 (Que.) Rev. Leg. 83, reversing Superior Court (Montreal), which had rendered a judgment in favor of the plaintiff
109. Johnstone v. Pedlar, (1921) 90 L.J.P.C. 181 (Eng.)
110. McFarland v. The Queen, (1882) S.C.R. 216
111. R.S.Q. 1950, c. 307, c. 33
112. R.S.O. 1950, c. 228, s. 41
113. R. v. Baker [1929] 1 D.L.R. 785 (Sup. Ct.)
114. Rex v. Giardine (1939) 71 Can. C.C. 295 (Ont. Co. Ct.)
115. See also R. v. Greisman (1926), 46 Can. C.C. 172 (Ont. C.A.), which quoted at

length from R. v. Bateman (post, note 114): "I think the great weight of authority goes to show that there will be no criminal liability unless there is gross negligence, or wanton misconduct" (p. 177). See also *Martin's Criminal Code.* § 191

116. Rex v. Batemen (1925) 19 Cr. App. R. 8, [1925] L.J.K.B. 792 (general practitioner charged with the manslaughter of a woman by tearing out her uterus in mistake for the placenta)

117. St. Onge v. Bernier (1932) 70 C.S. 205 (Que.)

118. Regina v. Judge [1957] 118 C.C.C. 410

119. *Martin's Criminal Code,* § 230; *Criminal Code,* s.c., 1953-54, Sec. 231 (2)

120. Agnew v. Jobson (1877) 13 Cox C.C. 625 (Eng.)

121. *Martin's Criminal Code,* Par. 192, 193

122. A summary of the attempts to control the importation and distribution of narcotics in Canada is found in Curran: *Canada's Food and Drug Laws.* New York, 1953, p. 76 ff.

123. Opium and Narcotic Drug Act, R.S.C. 1952, c. 201, in the most recent codification

124. Section 5 of the statute sets forth the penalties for violations. The penalties are a fine not exceeding $1000 and not less than $200 or imprisonment for a term not exceeding 18 months, or both fine and imprisonment

125. Morelli v. Rex, (1932) 52 B.R. 440 (Que.) 58 Can. CC 120, [1932] 3 D.L.R. 611, 28 Can. Abr. 991 followed. See also Re Au Chung Lam. 17 M.P.R. 254, 81 Can. C.C. 27, [1944] 1 D.L.R. 742 (N.S.C.A.). Leave to appeal refused, [1944] S.C.R. 136 *sub nom* Au Chung Lam, alias Ou Lim v. Rex, 81 Can. C.C. 113, [1944] 2 D.L.R. 401

126. R. v. Ryan (1947) 20 M.P.R. 320 (N.S. Sup. Ct.)

127. Lavellée v. Rex, (1936) 60 B.R. 349 (Que.), 66 Can. C.C. 101, [1936] 3 D.L.R. 570 (C.A.)

128. Fidler and Gray: *op. cit. supra.* note 24, pp. 45-46, on rules for dispensing narcotics

129. Sec. 237(1), formerly section 303 in the pre-1953-54 Code. Subsection 2 of this section makes it criminal for a pregnant woman to procure her own miscarriage

130. Section 238

131. R. v. Goodhall (1846) 1 Den. 187, 169 Eng. Rep. 205, indictment in England under 1 Vict. c. 85, prototype of the Canadian statute. It turned out that the woman was not pregnant, but this was held to be immaterial

132. R. v. Pettibone [1918] 2 W.W.R. 806, 809 (Alta.). See also R. v. Cramp (1880) 14 Cox C.C. 401, for interesting reasoning of Chief Justice Coleridge

133. R. v. Azoulay (1952-53), 15 C.R. 181 (Sup. Ct. Canada)

134. *In re* Sample [1955] 3 D.L.R. 199 (Sask. C.A.)

135. Robins v. National Trust Co., Ltd. [1927] 2 D.L.R. 97, A.C. 515, 56 O.L.R. 46

136. See Meredith: Insanity as a Criminal Defence – A Conflict of Views. 25 *Can. Bar Rev.,* 251 (1947); and Stevenson: Insanity as a Criminal Defence: The Psychiatric Viewpoint. 25 *Can. Bar Rev.,* 731 (1947)

137. Haines: Courts and Doctors. 30 *Can. Bar Rev.,* 483 (1952)

138. R.S.C. 1927, c. 59, s. 5(1); R.S.O. 1950, c. 119, s. 7(1)

139. C. 31, s. 5, amended by 1898, c. 53, s. 1 and by 1901, c. 36, s. 11; now R.S.C. 1927, c. 59, s. 5. See also MacRae: *Evidence,* p. 318

140. See the interesting discussion of the scope of s. 5(2) of the Canada Evidence Act and its relationship to the Quebec Code of Civil Procedure, art. 331, in Silberberg v. Caron, [1951] C.S. 131 (Que.); Requérants ex parte Lévesque et Autres, [1951] C.S. 140 (Que.). The Canada Evidence Act, s. 5(2), does not extend to incriminating documents produced by a witness under compulsion of a provincial statute

141. Hepenstal v. Merritt, (1895) 33 N.B. 91 (N.B. Sup. Ct.), affirming 25 S.C.R. 150, in which a nurse was permitted at trial to say that in her opinion a urinary trouble with which a child was affected resulted from an accident which was the subject of the suit

142. On the subject of the nurse and doctor as witness, see Haines: Courts and Doctors. 30 *Can. Bar Rev.,* 483 (1952)

Index

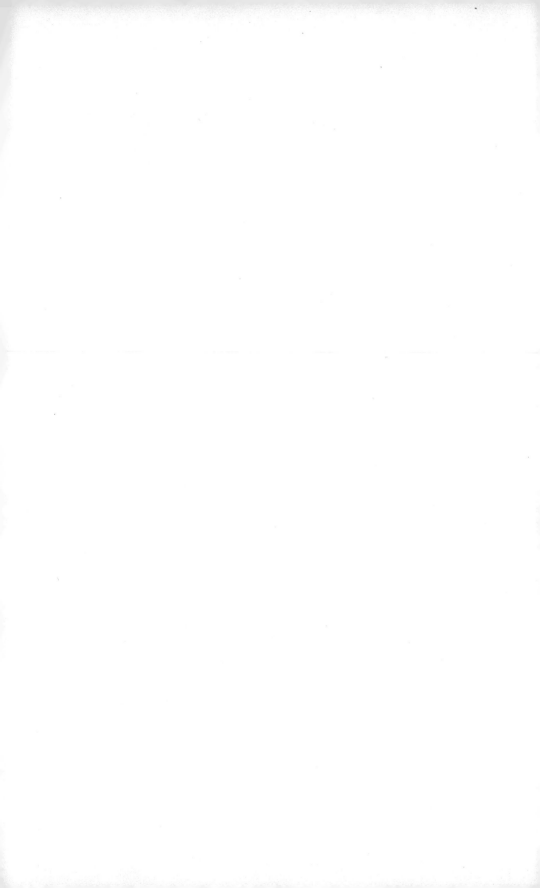